# Urodynamics Made Easy

Christopher R Chapple
and
Scott A MacDiarmid

W.B. Saunders Company

London . Edinburgh . New York . Philadelphia . St Louis . Sydney . Toronto . 2000

WB SAUNDERS
An imprint of Harcourt Publishers Limited

© Harcourt Publishers 2000

🅦 is a registered trademark of Harcourt Limited

The right of C. R. Chapple and S. A. MacDiarmid to be identified as authors of this work has been asserted by them in accordance with the Copyright, Designs and Patents Act 1988.

First published 2000

ISBN 0-4430-5463-0

**British Library Cataloguing in Publication Data**
A catalogue record for this book is available from the British Library

**Library of Congress Cataloguing in Publication Data**
A catalog record for this book is available from the Library of Congress

**Note**
Medical knowledge is constantly changing. As new information becomes available, changes in treatment, procedures, equipment and the use of drugs become necessary. The editors/authors/contributors and the publishers have, as far as it is possible, taken care to ensure that the information given in this text is accurate and up-to-date. However, readers are strongly advised to confirm that the information, especially with regard to drug usuage, complies with the latest legislation and standards of practice.

Commissioning Editor: Sue Hodgson
Design Direction: Ian Spick
Production Manager: Mark Sanderson

The publisher's policy is to use **paper manufactured from sustainable forests**

Typeset by IMH (Cartrif), Loanhead, Scotland
Printed and bound in Spain by Grafos S.A., Arte sobre papel, Barcelona.

# Contents

# Preface

This book aims to dispel the image that urodynamics is a complex subject. Urodynamics is not an esoteric subject of limited applicability and requiring complex equipment that is best confined to the 'ivory towers'. The basic principles of urodynamics are simple and in most cases complex investigation is unnecessary.

Factors that have fostered the popular erroneous image that urodynamics is complex are:
- first, the application of theoretical physics to the subject – although producing useful models on which to base further research, this is of limited use to the practising clinician; it is, however, useful to consider the urinary tract as a series of conduits within which urine movement is dictated by the pressures acting upon them and their resistance to flow, with specific sphincteric mechanisms acting as zones of variable resistance;
- second, the use of jargon terms that have tended to complicate and obscure otherwise logical and straightforward concepts – to clarify this the official terminology relating to urodynamics (presented in the format specified by the International Continence Society) is reviewed in this book.

This guide outlines the principles and practice of urodynamics in the routine clinical management of patients. Although the 'bladder is an unreliable witness' producing a variety of nonspecific symptoms, improvements in urodynamic techniques and electronic equipment over the past 20 years allow widespread use of objective investigations to clarify these symptoms.

Urodynamics is the study of pressure and flow relationships during the storage and transport of urine within the urinary tract. In routine practice most urodynamic investigations are focused on the lower urinary tract to:
- investigate bladder filling and voiding function;
- accurately define bladder storage disorders; and
- assess the severity of voiding dysfunction.

Upper tract urodynamics is usually carried out in specialist units.

The first edition of this book was compiled with Tim Christmas who due to other commitments has been unable to participate in the authorship of this edition. This role has been assumed by Scott MacDiarmid a urologist working in the USA who has a particular interest in urodynamics and functional assessment of the lower urinary tract. He has expanded the scope of clinical practice covered in this book to increase its usefulness to the practising clinician.

CRC December 1999

# Foreword

Although history and physical examination are sufficient to diagnose many patients, others require more sophisticated assessment such as urodynamic testing. Fueled by an array of refined electronic devices, the field of urodynamics has expanded in parallel with increases in knowledge about dysfunction of the lower urinary tract. Adequately treating incontinence, voiding difficulties, and other bladder disorders, in patients of all ages and either sex, may require consultation with various specialists. Many of these specialists may be unfamiliar, or have only limited knowledge, of the beneficial role urodynamics can play in the overall evaluation and management of their patients.

This book takes seriously the challenging task of educating physicians, and it provides basic information that can make "urodynamics easy," in a clear, concise, yet thorough style. The ten chapters comprehensibly cover the main topics of interest. Each chapter offers a section outlining the rationale for current medical or surgical therapies and includes practical examples, illustrations, flow charts, and visually appealing summary tables. By enhancing the text with full-color artwork, we hope readers will be able to assess key points more clearly. Additionally, along with relevant concepts on good urodynamic practice, an update is provided on new equipment and tests.

Not surprisingly, this second edition builds on the success of the first – a tribute to the authors' experience and recognized didactic talent in the field of urodynamics. The editors belong to a generation whose training included routine urodynamic testing and have learned from years of experience its unique and pivotal role in modern urology. This book will be an invaluable reference not only to students and residents but practitioners, gynecologists, general surgeons, and pediatricians in everyday practice.

Philippe Zimmern, M.D.
Associate Professor of Urology
Helen J. and Robert S. Strauss Professor in Urology

# Acknowledgements

We are particularly grateful to Nicholas Bryan and Karen Glass for their help and comments, particularly relating to the sections on pregnancy and ambulatory urodynamics. Our thanks also go to the International Continence Society for its permission to reproduce figures and definitions from its documents on standardisation.

# Chapter 1 | Use of urodynamics in clinical practice for evaluating the lower urinary tract

## INTRODUCTION

The lower urinary tract comprises the bladder and urethra. It should be considered as a single functioning vesicourethral unit that is required to:
* store urine adequately;
* empty efficiently.

Any disturbance of these fundamental tasks can result in urinary dysfunction and symptoms including:
* storage symptoms of frequency/urgency;
* incontinence;
* voiding symptoms (c.f. slow stream);
* urinary retention.

The bladder tends to be an 'unreliable witness', its symptoms often being nonspecific, neither revealing the diagnosis nor paralleling the severity of any underlying disorder.

Clinical evaluation of patients who have both storage and voiding dysfunction is based on the findings of:
* an in-depth history and physical examination;
* appropriate laboratory studies;
* when clinically indicated, endoscopy and radiography – provide useful structural information; and
* if appropriate, urodynamic studies.

### URODYNAMICS IN PRACTICE

Urodynamic studies
* provide the only objective functional tests of bladder and urethral function
* are a valuable adjunct in the investigation of patients who have lower urinary tract dysfunction

When properly selected and accurately interpreted, urodynamic studies improve diagnostic capability and are useful in formulating treatment strategies, educating patients, and improving therapeutic outcome.

Urodynamic studies should only be interpreted in conjunction with the clinical presentation. In most cases the indications for urodynamic investigation are evident and its use plays a vital role in the modern clinical practice of urology, gynaecology, and associated specialties. Just occasionally interpretation is not straightforward.

It is essential to use standardized jargon when practising urodynamics to allow accurate exchange and comparison of information for clinical and experimental purposes, so the official terminology suggested by the International Continence Society is defined and used throughout this book.

# URINARY INCONTINENCE

## In women
Women who have a history of pure stress urinary incontinence associated with urethrovesical hypermobility and no previous history may not necessarily require urodynamic evaluation before surgery for stress incontinence. However, a diagnosis made on the basis of history alone will not exclude detrusor overactivity in up to 25% of cases. Urodynamic assessment is therefore an important preoperative requisite for many women who present with stress incontinence, particularly those who have other associated abnormalities or risk factors that may complicate the presentation and influence treatment. These include patients who have:
- marked overactive bladder symptoms (mixed stress and urge incontinence);
- recurrent incontinence following previous surgery;
- associated or suspected neurological disease;
- dysfunctional voiding with high postvoid residual urine volumes;
- urge incontinence not responding to behavioural and pharmacological management.

## In men
Most cases of male urinary incontinence are due to either:
- overactive bladder;
- neuropathic bladder;
- prostatectomy; or
- overflow incontinence.

Urodynamics forms the cornerstone for evaluating male voiding dysfunction. Indications for urodynamics include:
- any type of urinary incontinence;
- diagnosing urethral sphincter insufficiency;
- obstructive voiding combined with marked urinary frequency and urgency;

- chronic retention;
- recurrent symptoms after previous surgery;
- patients who have a history of documented neurological disease or possible neuropathy (e.g. diabetes mellitus);
- younger patients (<55 years of age).

## BLADDER OUTLET OBSTRUCTION

### In men

Obstructive voiding symptoms can be caused by a variety of disorders including:
- bladder outlet obstruction (BOO) secondary to benign prostatic hyperplasia (BPH), urethral stricture, bladder neck dyssynergia;
- poor detrusor contractility;
- functional obstruction from detrusor–sphincter dyssynergia.

Urodynamics can help in diagnosing the underlying pathological process by appropriate use of uroflowmetry, pressure–flow studies, and videourodynamics.

Uroflowmetry combined with a postvoiding ultrasound residual volume is an excellent screening test for symptomatic men who have BOO. A normal flow rate does not exclude obstruction due to compensatory bladder changes (in up to 15% of cases) and pressure–flow studies are required for diagnosis. Other patients who fall into the groups listed above would also benefit from pressure–flow urodynamics.

## NEUROPATHIC BLADDER

All symptomatic patients who have neuropathic bladder dysfunction should undergo urodynamics and preferably videourodynamics to:
- characterize the detrusor and sphincteric abnormality accurately;
- identify patients who are at risk of developing renal damage from their lower tract abnormality.

More sophisticated electrophysiological studies are useful in diagnosing neuropathic bladder in selected patients. The most commonly studied patients are those who have:
- multiple sclerosis;
- stroke;
- diabetes mellitus;
- Parkinson's disease;
- spinal cord injury.

## PAEDIATRIC VOIDING DYSFUNCTION

Urodynamics plays a minor role in the evaluation of otherwise healthy children who have urinary incontinence and abnormal voiding patterns. Sometimes it is used to confirm a diagnosis of bladder overactivity in school-aged children who have urinary frequency and urge incontinence that fails to respond to therapy.

Children who have isolated enuresis do not always have urodynamic abnormalities; conversely a history of childhood enuresis is commonly seen in patients who are diagnosed as having detrusor instability later in life.

Urodynamics is mandatory in the evaluation of children who have:
- acquired functional voiding disorders including Hinman's syndrome;
- spinal abnormalities;
- neuropathic bladder following spinal cord injury.

| **Structure and function of the urinary tract**

## INTRODUCTION

The urinary tract consists of two mutually dependent components:
- upper tract (kidneys and ureters);
- lower tract (bladder and urethra).

This provides a highly sophisticated system of conduits that converts the continuous involuntary production of urine by the kidneys into the intermittent, consciously controlled voiding of urine (micturition) in appropriate circumstances.

The upper tracts function as a low-pressure distensible conduit with intrinsic peristalsis, which transports urine from the nephrons via the ureters to the bladder. The vesicoureteric mechanism protects the nephrons from damage that might arise from retrograde transmission of back pressure or infection from the bladder.

## THE URINARY BLADDER

The bladder has two main functions:
- collection and low-pressure storage of urine;
- expulsion of urine at an appropriate time and in an appropriate place.
  Histologically it is made up of three layers:
- an outer adventitial connective tissue layer;
- a middle smooth muscle coat (detrusor muscle), comprising a functional syncytium of interlacing muscle bundles;
- an innermost lining comprised of transitional cell epithelium providing an elastic barrier that is impervious to urine (Figure 2.1).

### Innervation
The detrusor muscle is controlled by the autonomic nervous system and is richly innervated by three groups of nerves:
- the principal population is comprised of presumptive cholinergic nerves (identified by their content of the enzyme acetylcholinesterase and demonstrated by the use of electron microscopy to lie in close apposition to muscle cells) – by releasing the neurotransmitter acetylcholine they provide the major motor control of the detrusor muscle;
- the sympathetic innervation comprises a sparse distribution of noradrenergic neurones, which occur in greatest concentration towards

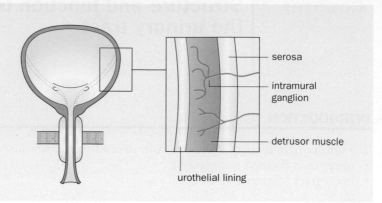

**Figure 2.1 Structure of the bladder wall.** The bladder wall is comprised of three layers and has a rich innervation of cholinergic, adrenergic, and nonadrenergic noncholinergic sensorimotor nerves. Intramural ganglia allow extensive neural interaction.

the bladder base and are thought to be of principal importance in controlling the vasculature;
- the third population of nonadrenergic noncholinergic (NANC) sensorimotor nerves contains a variety of putative neurotransmitters (principally peptides), which can be identified by immunofluorescent techniques – their precise role in controlling the human bladder is not clear.

The close juxtaposition of these neural populations allows them to interact. To facilitate this there are potential neural links via ganglia at every level from the spinal cord to the target organs (prostate, bladder, sphincters), in particular between the parasympathetic and sympathetic nervous systems.

The spinal segments S2–S4 act via efferent parasympathetic cholinergic neurones to initiate and maintain detrusor contraction. Damage to these spinal segments abolishes the micturition reflex.

After leaving the sacral foramina, the pelvic splanchnic nerves containing the parasympathetic innervation to the bladder pass lateral to the rectum to enter the inferior hypogastric or pelvic plexus. They are joined by the hypogastric nerve containing efferent sympathetic nerve fibres originating from the spinal cord segments T10–L2. When combined they form a plexus at the base of the bladder.

It has been suggested that:
- the pelvic nerves provide the main afferent pathway of the micturition reflex – there is now increasing evidence to suggest that the urothelium and its associated afferent innervation has an important role in the normal control of micturition;

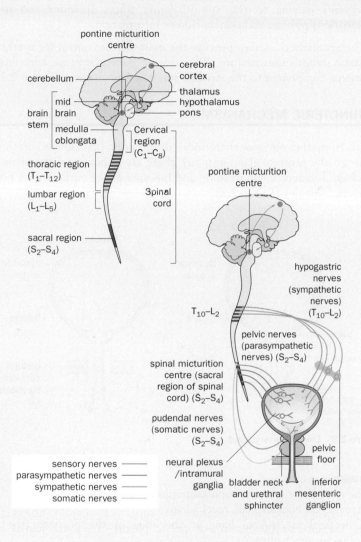

**Figure 2.2  Neural control of the lower urinary tract.** There is extensive interaction within the spinal cord and in paravesical and intramural bladder ganglia (not shown).

- sympathetic neuronal pathways in the hypogastric nerves (innervating the trigone) passing to the spinothalamic tracts (bladder and urethral sensation) provide additional afferent information.

The sympathetic nerves provide the main motor control for urethral and prostatic smooth musculature. The somatic pudendal nerve contributes an additional component to the striated sphincter mechanism (Figure 2.2).

## SPHINCTERIC MECHANISMS

Apart from the obvious anatomical differences (the longer urethra and presence of a prostate gland in men), there are important differences in the histological structure, innervation, and function of the outflow tract between males and females (Figure 2.3).

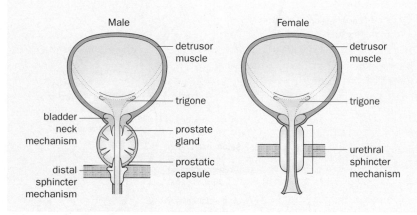

**Figure 2.3   Lower urinary tract.**

### In males
In the male there are two important sphincteric mechanisms:
- a proximal 'bladder neck mechanism';
- a urethral mechanism lying at the apex of the prostate (the 'distal sphincter mechanism').

The male bladder neck is a powerful sphincter subserving both the urinary and genital roles, the latter function being of primary importance in preventing retrograde ejaculation.

The distal sphincteric mechanism is also extremely important as evidenced by its ability to maintain continence even when the bladder neck has been rendered totally incompetent by bladder neck incision or prostatectomy. Conversely in patients who have a damaged distal urethral sphincter (e.g. as in pelvic fracture-associated urethral disruption) continence is maintained by the bladder neck mechanism.

## In females
The female bladder neck is a far weaker structure than the male bladder neck and can be incompetent, even in nulliparous young women. Urinary continence in women usually relies upon the integrity of the intrinsic urethral sphincteric mechanism. Damage to the innervation of the urethral sphincter (in particular the pudendal nerve) by obstetric trauma predisposes to urinary stress incontinence.

## Ultrastructural findings
The functional observations for the sphincteric mechanisms are mirrored by the ultrastructural findings.

### Bladder neck
Ultrastructurally, the bladder neck:
* in males consists of two muscular layers – a powerful inner layer of muscle bundles arranged in a circular orientation containing a rich adrenergic sympathetic nerve supply and an outer layer contiguous with the detrusor muscle and receiving both a cholinergic and adrenergic innervation;
* in females is poorly defined with the muscle fibres having a mainly longitudinal orientation and the predominant innervation being cholinergic.

### Urethral sphincter mechanism
This is composed of intrinsic urethral smooth muscle and extrinsic striated muscle components and:
* in females it extends throughout the proximal two-thirds of the urethra, being most developed in the middle one-third of the urethra, particularly dorsally;
* in males it is localized to the prostatic apex.

### Extrinsic component of the urethral sphincter
The efferent innervation of the striated muscle of the extrinsic component of the urethral sphincter arises predominantly from cell bodies lying in a specific area of the sacral anterior horn known as Onuf's nucleus. Various aspects of the innervation of this sphincter are controversial – not only the neural pathways involved, but also the relative contribution of somatic and autonomic nerves. The limited knowledge available suggests that the pudendal nerve transmits urethral mucosal sensation.

### Prostate gland
The prostate is made up of smooth muscle and glandular tissue, the proportion of smooth muscle being increased in benign prostatic hyperplasia. This muscle

is controlled by the sympathetic nervous system, which acts by releasing noradrenaline onto $\alpha_{1A}$ adrenoceptors located on prostatic smooth muscle cells.

## MICTURITION REFLEXES

Before considering the clinical investigation and treatment of disorders of micturition it is first essential to consider the neural mechanisms controlling urinary tract function. Although most contemporary knowledge is based on studies with experimental animals, it is difficult and often misleading to relate the findings from such animal models directly to man. However, data for humans are limited as they can only be obtained from studying clearly defined clinical syndromes and isolated spinal cord lesions.

The pioneering neurophysiologist, Barrington, initially described five reflexes associated with micturition in the cat, to which he added a further two after further study. Two of these reflexes had reflex centres in supraspinal sites (medulla and pons) and caused strong and sustained contractions. He considered that these were essential for normal micturition because bladder contraction and urethral relaxation are not coordinated after experimentally produced high spinal transection. The remaining five reflexes appeared to be confined to the spinal cord. More recently it has been proposed that many interrelated reflexes act upon the sacral micturition centre exerting both excitatory and inhibitory effects.

## URINE STORAGE AND VOIDING

Urine storage and voiding are two interrelated yet distinct phases of lower urinary tract function.

The bladder and urethra possess intrinsic tone produced by the muscle and connective tissue they contain. At rest, the urethral tone keeps the walls in apposition and aids continence. During filling the walls of the bladder exhibit receptive relaxation (i.e. the vesical lumen expands without resulting in a concomitant rise in intravesical pressure). The extent to which a change in volume ($\delta V$) occurs in relation to a change in intravesical pressure ($\delta P$) is known as the bladder compliance ($\delta V/\delta P$). Factors that contribute to this property are:
- the passive viscoelastic properties of the bladder; and
- the intrinsic ability of smooth muscle to maintain a constant tension over a wide range of stretch.

The other major factor controlling bladder filling is its neural control.

During bladder filling afferent activity from stretch receptors increases and passes via the posterior roots of the sacral cord and the lateral spinothalamic tracts to the brain, thereby mediating the desire to void. Activity within the striated component of the urethral sphincter is increased and local spinal reflex activity enhances the activity within striated muscles of the pelvic floor and sphincter to tighten up the bladder outlet mechanisms and so augment continence.

Important local factors facilitating bladder filling include both receptive relaxation and the passive viscoelastic properties of the bladder wall. Conditions that contribute to poor bladder compliance and detrusor instability (see pp. 110–115) include:

- abnormal bladder morphology resulting from collagenous infiltration, hypertrophy, or altered muscle structure (e.g. obstructed bladder); and
- abnormal detrusor smooth muscle behaviour, either primary or secondary to neural dysfunction.

### Initiation and control of voiding

Once a threshold level of filling has been achieved (which will depend upon circumstances and vary between individuals), increasing afferent activity will start to impinge on consciousness, resulting in awareness that the bladder is filling up. Except during infancy, in health there is complete volitional control over these reflex pathways and voiding will be initiated in appropriate circumstances. Micturition initiated by the cerebral cortex is likely to involve a complex series of bladder–brain stem reflexes.

During voiding:

- urethral relaxation precedes detrusor contraction;
- there is simultaneous relaxation of the pelvic floor muscles; and
- there is accompanying funnelling of the bladder neck.

The mechanism of these changes is not clear. It is likely that:

- increased activity within parasympathetic neurones results in removal of central inhibitory influences acting on the sacral centres; and
- voiding is initiated under the influence of pontine medullary centres.

There is therefore parasympathetically-controlled detrusor contraction associated with a corresponding relaxation of the urethra/prostate/bladder neck complex resulting from reciprocal nerve-mediated inhibition of the sympathetic nerve-mediated outflow.

In addition to these primary actions other important secondary events are:

- contraction of the diaphragm and anterior abdominal wall muscles;
- relaxation of the pelvic floor; and
- specific behavioural changes associated with voiding.

At the end of voiding the proximal urethra is closed in a retrograde fashion, the 'milkback' seen at videocystometry. Once these events have been completed, the sacral centres are re-inhibited by the cortex and the next filling cycle starts.

## VESICOURETHRAL FUNCTION

### Normal function

Normal function of the human lower urinary tract depends upon integrated coordination of the neural control of the bladder and outflow tract, for which an intact spinal cord is essential.

Under normal circumstances:
- bladder capacity is approximately 500 ml and the bladder empties, leaving no residual urine;
- males void at a pressure of 40–50 cm $H_2O$ and a maximum flow rate of 30–40 ml/s; and
- females void at a pressure of 30–40 cm $H_2O$ and a maximum flow rate of 40–50 ml/s.

The difference between males and females is a consequence of the higher outflow resistance exerted by the male urethra.

## Abnormal function

Disordered lower urinary tract function can result from:
- disruption of the normal peripheral or central nervous system (CNS) control mechanisms; and
- disordered bladder muscle function, either primary (of unknown aetiology) or secondary to an identifiable pathology such as prostatic-mediated bladder outflow obstruction.

### CLINICAL NOTES

- Patients who have disordered lower urinary tract function in routine clinical practice represent a heterogeneous collection for most of whom there is no identifiable neurological abnormality
- Some of these patients will have a primary neural or muscular disorder (e.g. primary idiopathic detrusor instability) in contrast to postobstructive secondary detrusor instability where the major aetiological factor is likely to be peripheral disruption of local neuromuscular function.

### Disruption of normal peripheral or central nervous system control mechanisms

A neurological classification is invaluable for counselling and can be of useful prognostic significance. Certain characteristic patterns – peripheral denervation, suprasacral spinal cord lesions, and cerebral (suprapontine) lesions – can be identified (see below).

### Peripheral denervation

The clinical picture of peripheral denervation depends upon the extent of denervation. Complete lesions decentralize the lower urinary tract and although ganglionic activity may persist, an acontractile bladder will result with an inactive urethra. Subsequent continence is governed by the functional competence of the bladder neck mechanism. The urethra has a fixed resistance and bladder emptying depends upon abdominal straining or manual compression. Partial lesions often result in detrusor hyperreflexia.

### Suprasacral spinal cord lesions

If the spinal cord is transected above the fifth lumbar segment, a 'cord bladder' develops. A principal feature of this lesion is loss of coordinated detrusor–sphincter behaviour, which results in simultaneous contraction of the detrusor and urethral sphincter (detrusor–sphincter dyssynergia). Sphincter contractions are not usually prolonged throughout the period of detrusor action, so there is intermittent voiding, but also urine retention. Voiding function can be particularly ineffective in people who have lesions of the thoracolumbar cord, and in these people low compliance is an important feature.

### Cerebral (suprapontine) lesions

Lesions of the midbrain rarely result in disturbances of continence and micturition. It is likely that this is due to:
- the bilateral representation of nuclei at this level; and
- the poor prognosis of patients who have extensive lesions.

Damage to the basal ganglia results in a reduced threshold for the transmission of impulses through the reticulospinal tracts controlling micturition. The typical picture is therefore of involuntary bladder contractions, which occur in people who have Parkinson's disease and following cerebrovascular thrombosis or haemorrhage.

Lesions of the cerebral cortex, in particular involving the inner surface of the cerebral hemispheres or the frontal cortex, can result in incontinence. It is felt that these patients lose the centrally mediated inhibition of the pontine voiding reflex resulting in involuntary bladder contractions and urge incontinence.

### CLINICAL NOTES

Many urinary disorders seen in clinical practice may have a neurological cause, but a classification based on specific abnormalities and in particular the site of a neurological lesion is not practical because:
- the aetiology and pathogenesis of many disorders is at present unclear;
- lesions are often difficult to locate and once located can be difficult to relate to the neurological signs (e.g. multiple sclerosis); and
- different lesions can produce identical functional changes in the lower urinary tract.

## DISORDERS OF THE LOWER URINARY TRACT

Disorders of the lower urinary tract can best be subdivided into:

- disorders of sensation; and
- disorders of motor function.

Each of these may affect:
- the detrusor muscle; or
- the sphincter-active bladder outflow tract (bladder neck mechanism, distal urethral sphincter mechanism, prostate).

The detrusor muscle and the sphincter-active bladder outflow tract may be normal, overactive or underactive.

## Disorders of sensation

These disorders represent an important poorly understood group of conditions where investigation is limited by:
- limited knowledge about the structural and physiological basis for the perception of sensation in the lower urinary tract; and
- the subjective nature of sensation.

Attempts to quantify sensation have included the use of objective or semi-objective tests for sensory function such as evoked potentials and electrical threshold studies.

At present disorders of sensation are usually assessed by asking the patient about voiding pattern and any discomfort felt, based on clinical questioning or cystometry.

Because most sensory disorders are idiopathic, diagnosis of such a disorder can only be considered after other vesical or urethral pathologies (tumour, stone, infection, abnormal detrusor function) have been excluded.

In general terms, sensation can be subdivided as normal, hypersensitive, hyposensitive, and absent.

### TERMINOLOGY: DISORDERS OF SENSATION

- **First sensation of filling:** very subjective; a variable and unreliable symptom
- **First desire to void:** can be difficult to interpret; very subjective
- **Strong desire to void:** indicates maximum bladder capacity and signals the end of bladder filling during cystometry
- **Pain:** pain during bladder filling or micturition is abnormal; its site and character should be noted, as well as the volume at which it occurred.

## Disorders of detrusor motor function

Cystometry is needed to assess detrusor function and not only may detrusor function differ during filling and voiding, but the classification may change between these two phases.

Detrusor function should be considered in the context of coexisting urethral function, but is often the primary cause of marked functional disruption.

Detrusor function may be:

- normal (stable);
- overactive;
- underactive (hypocontractile); or
- acontractile.

## TERMINOLOGY: DISORDERS OF DETRUSOR MOTOR FUNCTION

- **Stable detrusor function:** during filling bladder capacity increases in volume without a marked corresponding rise in pressure
- **Normal detrusor contractility:** normal voiding occurs as a result of a sustained detrusor contraction, which can be initiated and suppressed voluntarily and results in complete bladder emptying over a normal timespan; the magnitude of the recorded detrusor pressure rise depends upon outlet resistance
- **Overactive bladder:** a descriptive term that is applied to the combination in part or together of the lower urinary tract symptoms of urgency plus frequency, nocturia or urge incontinence
- **Overactive detrusor function:** involuntary detrusor contractions during bladder filling, either spontaneous or provoked by rapid filling (provocation cystometry), provocative tests (hand washing, heel bouncing, alteration in posture, exercise, or coughing)
- **Unstable detrusor:** detrusor that is objectively shown to contract either spontaneously or on provocation during the filling phase during an attempt to inhibit micturition; it may be asymptomatic and it occurs in the absence of a documented neurological disorder
- **Detrusor hyperreflexia:** detrusor hyperactivity in the presence of a documented neurological disorder
- **Detrusor instability:** detrusor hyperactivity in the absence of a documented neurological disorder
- **Normal compliance:** little or no rise in detrusor pressure during normal bladder filling; at present there are insufficient data to adequately define normal, high, and low compliance
- **Low compliance:** gradual rise in detrusor pressure during bladder filling; usually describes a poorly distensible bladder (e.g. a shrunken fibrotic bladder complicating interstitial cystitis or after radiotherapy); detrusor instability and hyperreflexia also may be associated with low compliance
- **Underactive (hypocontractile) detrusor function:** detrusor contraction during micturition is inadequate to empty the bladder

- **Acontractile detrusor:** no contractile activity on urodynamic investigation
- **Areflexic detrusor:** acontractility resulting from a neurological abnormality
- **Decentralized detrusor:** a specific type of areflexic detrusor that occurs with lesions of the conus medullaris or sacral nerve outflow, where the peripheral ganglia in the wall of the bladder are preserved and the peripheral nerves are therefore intact but 'decentralized'; characterized by involuntary intravesical pressure fluctuations of low amplitude, sometimes called 'autonomous waves'
- **Genuine stress incontinence:** is said to occur when there is demonstrable incontinence associated with a rise in intra-abdominal pressure in the absence of detrusor overactivity. It is due to intrinsic urethral sphincteric weakness.
- **Mixed incontinence:** is a situation where there is a combination of detrusor overactivity and urethral sphincteric weakness

## Bladder outflow tract dysfunction

The urethral closure mechanisms, including intrinsic urethral muscle and the sphincteric mechanisms (bladder neck and distal urethral) are best considered separately according to the phase of bladder function (either storage or voiding).

Urethral function during storage may be:
- normal – there is a positive urethral closure pressure that is sufficient to maintain continence in the presence of increased intra-abdominal pressure;
- incompetent – there is leakage, even in the absence of detrusor contraction; it may result fom damage to the urethra or the associated sphincteric mechanisms;
- underactive; or
- absent.

Urethral function during micturition may be:
- normal – the urethra opens to allow the bladder to be emptied;
- obstructive due to overactivity – the urethral closure mechanisms contract against a detrusor contraction or fail to open on attempted micturition – when this occurs in the absence of documented neurological disease it is known as 'dysfunctional voiding';
- obstructive due to a mechanical problem – this is uncommon in women, but is the most common cause of bladder outflow tract dysfunction in the male population, usually due to urethral stricture or prostatic enlargement; mechanical obstruction can arise as a consequence of anatomical factors (e.g. prostatic enlargement due to adenomatous hyperplasia) or neural control mechanisms (e.g. providing a functional

basis for the relief of obstruction by $\alpha_1$-adrenoceptor blockade of the prostate). In this context it is notable that in recent years it has been increasingly recognised that an important component of prostatic obstruction results from smooth muscle contraction within the pathologically enlarged prostate.

### Detrusor–urethral dyssynergia
In detrusor–urethral dyssynergia there is synchronous contraction of the detrusor and urethra. It can be subdivided depending upon the structures involved into detrusor–bladder neck dyssynergia and detrusor–sphincter dyssynergia.

### Detrusor–bladder neck dyssynergia
This refers to a detrusor contraction in the presence of incomplete bladder neck opening on micturition. It is not uncommon in the general population, and is a common cause of voiding dysfunction in younger males. It is thought to be a congenital abnormality, and commonly presents in the third and fourth decades of life.

### Detrusor–sphincter dyssynergia
Detrusor–sphincter dyssynergia (DSD) describes a detrusor contraction occurring at the same time as an involuntary contraction of the urethral or periurethral striated smooth muscle.

Obstructive overactivity of the striated urethral sphincter muscle may occur in the absence of detrusor contraction, but is not DSD. This condition is uncommon in the general population, it affects women in particular and is most commonly seen in association with polycystic ovary disease.

Detrusor–sphincter dyssynergia is usually associated with neurological disorders and the diagnosis needs to be treated with caution in the absence of a documented neurological deficit.

## INTRODUCTION

Urinary continence during bladder filling, urine storage in the bladder, and the efficiency of subsequent voiding all depend upon accurate coordination of the opposing forces of:
- detrusor contraction; and
- urethral closure pressure.

Symptomatic evaluation of urinary tract dysfunction is difficult because the bladder often proves to be an 'unreliable witness', not only because of subjective bias, but also because there is considerable overlap between the symptoms for different disorders. Urodynamic techniques are objective investigations developed to clarify these symptoms. The term urodynamics encompasses a variety of complementary techniques of varying complexity (Figure 3.1). Their use needs to be tailored to each individual case.

This book provides a practical approach to the use of urodynamics, particularly for investigation of the lower urinary tract. Volume voided charts, pad testing, the use of postvoiding residuals, cystometry, and videocystometry are therefore discussed in more detail than other techniques. Urethral pressure profilometry is usually not necessary, particularly if videocystometry is used, because it is rather inaccurate, but is discussed in some detail because it is widely used. Neurophysiology is mentioned, but is a research tool. Upper tract urodynamics is a useful modality for highly selected cases.

In most cases there are clear indications for urodynamic investigation and its application is essential to the modern practice of urology, gynaecology, and any specialties dealing with the management of lower urinary tract dysfunction.

It is essential to use standardized jargon for urodynamic investigation to allow accurate exchange and comparison of information for both clinical and experimental purposes. The official terminology suggested by the International Continence Society is reviewed throughout the chapter.

### Exclude urinary tract infections first

Urinary tract infections (UTIs) are an uncommon cause of incontinence and should always be checked for before urodynamic investigation because:
- a UTI will aggravate any existing urinary symptoms; and
- the presence of a UTI can invalidate the results of urodynamics. The filling cystometrogram may falsely demonstrate bladder instability and in some

| Urodynamic techniques | |
|---|---|
| **Complexity of technique** | **Technique** |
| Simple | Volume voided charts |
| | Pad testing |
| | Flow rate |
| | Ultrasound cystodynamogram |
| | Intravenous urodynamogram |
| | Cystometry |
| | Videocystometrography |
| Complex | Urethral pressure measurement |
| | Ambulatory urodynamics |
| | Neurophysiological investigation |
| | Upper tract urodynamics (Whitaker test) |

Figure 3.1   Urodynamic techniques.

cases, loss of bladder compliance. The effects of asymptomatic bacteriurea on cystometry is unknown.

Confirmation of recurrent UTIs may alter the type and priority of investigations performed.

## VOLUME VOIDED CHARTS

The urodynamic value of the simple voided volume chart is often overlooked – an important omission because it provides a natural volumetric urodynamic record of bladder function (Figure 3.2).

The volume–frequency chart is a simple noninvasive tool used in the evaluation of patients who have voiding dysfunction, particularly those who have increased urinary frequency and incontinence. It helps to:
- define the severity of symptoms; and
- add objectivity to the history.

## Volume/Frequency chart

Week Commencing:  /   /

| | Monday | | Tuesday | | Wednesday | | Thursday | | Friday | | Saturday | | Sunday | |
|---|---|---|---|---|---|---|---|---|---|---|---|---|---|---|
| | In | Out | In | Out | In | Out | In | Out | In | Out | In | Out | In | Out |
| 6am | 300 | | | | 350 | | | | | | 200 | | 190 | |
| 7am | | | 200 | | | | 250 | | 350 | | 100 | | | 170 |
| 8am | | 50 | | | | 150 | | | | 250 | | 190 | | |
| 9am | 250 | 150 | | 100 | | | 150 | | | | | | | |
| 10am | | | | | 150 | | | 200 | | | | | 100 | |
| 11am | 175 | 100 | | | 175 | | | | 200 | | 180 | | | |
| 12.00 | | | 250 | | | 100 | | | | | | 150 | | 130 |
| 1pm | | | | | | | 200 | | | 200 | | | | |
| 2pm | 190 | W | | 130 | 150 | | | 175 | | | | | | 270 |
| 3pm | | | | | | W | | | 100 | W | 270 | | | |
| 4pm | | | | | | | | W | | | | | | |
| 5pm | 300 | 200 | | | | 150 | 200 | | | 150 | | W | | W |
| 6pm | | | | 190 | 200 | | | | | | | | | |
| 7pm | | 75 | | W | | 100 | | 150 | | | 100 | | 180 | |
| 8pm | | | | | | 100 | | | 200 | 175 | | | | |
| 9pm | 150 | 100 | | | | | | | | | | | 120 | |
| 10pm | | | 150 | | | | | | 175 | | 190 | | | 175 |
| 11pm | | | | | | | 100 | | | 100 | | | | |
| 12.00 | | | | 50 | | W | | 100 | | | 100 | | | |
| 1am | | | | | | | | | | | | | 100 | |
| 2am | | W | | | | | | | | W | | W | | 120 |
| 3am | | | | | | 120 | | | | | | | | |
| 4am | | | | | | | | | | | | | | |
| 5am | | | 150 | | | | | | | | | | | |
| Waking | 6am | | 7.45am | | 7.30am | | 7.00am | | 6.30am | | 7.45am | | 7.40am | |
| Retiring | 12.30am | | 11.30pm | | 12.51am | | Midnight | | Midnight | | 12.30am | | 11.30pm | |
| Pad usage | 3 | | 1 | | 2 | | 4 | | 3 | | 5 | | 2 | |

**Figure 3.2  Volume voided chart.** Key: Patients should fill in frequency of voiding, indicating time of going to bed and getting up to allow calculation of nocturia. Episodes of incontinence should be documented by the use of a (W) in the shaded areas, as well as number of pads. Additional information which can be collected is the volume of fluid intake and voided volumes.

## BLADDER RE-TRAINING PROGRAMME

In order to bring your bladder problem under control you must learn to stretch your bladder. Stretching your bladder will help to control leakage and you can do this by trying to hold on for as long as possible before passing water.

It is important that you **do not** restrict your fluid intake.

- When you get the feeling, that you want to pass urine, **hold on for as long as you possibly can**.
- At first this will be difficult but as you persevere it will become easier.
- Sitting on a hard seat may help you to hold on to your urine for longer.
- If you wake up at night, try to hold on if you can; if possible, turn over and go back to sleep.
- If you have been prescribed tablets to help you pass your urine less frequently take them regularly as directed.
- You should aim to reduce the frequency with which you pass urine to 5 or 6 times in 24 hours.

**Remember**

You are trying to stretch your bladder so that it will hold more urine. Although you may find this difficult at first, with practice it will get easier.

Increased urinary frequency secondary to high urinary output can be readily diagnosed and differentiated from physiological nocturnal diuresis. A record of fluid intake helps in identifying an easily treatable cause of urinary frequency.

The average maximum voided volume represents the patient's functional capacity and knowing what this volume is prevents overfilling of the bladder during cystometry:

- a normal bladder fills to a volume that approximates its functional capacity and the chart records a series of sizeable (300–500 ml) and fairly consistent volumes; and
- an unstable bladder contracts at variable degrees of distension before full capacity, erroneously informing the patient that it is full, resulting in urinary frequency and low and varying voided volumes.

Volume–frequency charts also provide important feedback to the practitioner and patient so that they can objectively evaluate the effectiveness of any therapy.

## URODYNAMICS IN PRACTICE: VOLUME VOIDED CHARTS

To produce a volume voided chart the patient is instructed to:
- record fluid intake; and
- the time and volume of each void for 3–5 days (Figure 3.2).

Episodes of incontinence, the use of pads and episodes of urgency should also be recorded.

### Bladder drill
Patients are instructed to:
- hold on to their urine for a fixed time, such as 1 hour;
- then void, recording the volume voided and incontinent episodes; and
- gradually increase the time between voids until an acceptable voiding pattern is achieved.

### Practical points
Symptoms and the volume voided chart often vary considerably from week to week if there is sensory frequency resulting from:
- a hypersensitive bladder due to urine infection, trigonitis, or a condition such as interstitial cystitis; and
- a hypersensitive urethra – the urethral syndrome.

It is essential not to base therapy on the results of such investigation alone; in particular it is essential to  exclude other aetiologies for the bladder symptoms such as neoplasia, carcinoma *in situ*, or intravesical stones before proceeding with therapy.

### Comment
The volume voided chart can provide information that is helpful in both assessing and treating bladder dysfunction. It is particularly useful for providing biofeedback during bladder retraining drills commonly used in patients with small volume frequency and urge incontinence (see above). The results must not be overinterpreted, but should be used in combination with other forms of urodynamic and urological assessment.

## PAD TESTING

A subjective asssessment of incontinence is often difficult to interpret and does not reliably indicate the degree of abnormality. Not all patients who complain of urinary incontinence are incontinent during a cystometric examination. Pad testing is a simple noninvasive objective method for detecting and quantifying urine leakage.

## Quantification of urine loss

To obtain a representative result, especially for those who have variable or intermittent urinary incontinence, the test period should be as long as possible in circumstances that approximate to those of everyday life and conducted in a standardized fashion.

### URODYNAMICS IN PRACTICE: PAD TESTING

The International Continence Society has suggested the following guidelines:
- The test should occupy a 1-hour period during which a series of standard activities are carried out
- The test can be extended by further 1-hour periods if the result of the first 1-hour test is not considered to be representative by either the patient or the investigator; alternatively the test can be repeated after filling the bladder to a defined volume
- The total amount of urine lost during the test period is determined by weighing a collecting device such as a nappy, absorbent pad, or condom appliance (ensure that the collecting device has adequate capacity)
- A nappy or pad should be worn inside waterproof underpants or should have a waterproof backing
- Immediately before the test begins the collecting device is weighed to the nearest gram (g)

**Typical test schedule**
- Test is started without the patient voiding
- Preweighed collecting device (pad) is put on and first 1-hour test period begins
- Patient drinks 500 ml sodium-free liquid within a short period (maximum 15 min), then sits or rests
- Patient walks for 30 min, including stair climbing equivalent to one flight up and down
- For remaining period the patient performs the following activities: standing up from sitting, 10 times; coughing vigorously, 10 times; running on the spot for 1 min; bending to pick up small object from floor, 5 times; washes hands in running water for 1 min
- At the end of the 1-hour test the collecting device is removed and weighed
- If the test is regarded as representative the subject voids and the volume is recorded, otherwise the test is repeated preferably without voiding
- If the collecting device becomes saturated or filled during the test it should be removed and weighed, and replaced by a fresh device
- The activity programme may be modified according to the patient's physical ability

## Practical points
### Interpretation
The total weight of urine lost during the test period is taken to be equal to the gain in weight of the collecting device(s). An increase in weight of the pad of less than 1 g in 1 hour is not considered to be a sign of incontinence because a weight gain of up to 1 g may be due to weighing errors, sweating, or vaginal discharge. Evaporation is not important.

The test should not be performed during a menstrual period and patients may influence the test result by voiding voluntarily.

A negative result should be interpreted with caution; the test may need to be repeated or supplemented with a more prolonged test.

The quantitative reproducibility of the 1-hour pad test is relatively poor. Substantial variations from the usual test schedule should be recorded so that the same schedule can be used on subsequent occasions.

### Voiding
In principle patients should not void during the test period. If they experience urgency, they should be persuaded to postpone voiding and to perform as many of the activities listed for the last 15–30 min of the test as possible to detect leakage. Before voiding the collection device is removed for weighing.

If voiding cannot be postponed the test is terminated. The voiding volume and duration of the test should be recorded. The results for patients who are unable to complete the test may require separate analysis or the test may be repeated after rehydration.

### Normal values
The hourly pad weight increase in continent women varies from 0.0 to 2.1 g/hour, averaging 0.26 g/hour. With the 1-hour International Continence Society pad test, the upper limit (99% confidence limit) has been found to be 1.4 g/hour.

### Home pad test
Home pad tests lasting 24–48 hours are superior to 1-hour tests in detecting urinary incontinence. The normal upper limit for a 24-hour test is 8 g. Although longer duration tests are better screening tests for incontinence they are less practical and more cumbersome. The pads must be stored in an airtight container before and after use to prevent evaporation.

### Variations to test procedure
Colouration of the urine with oral pyridium before pad testing can help differentiate between vaginal discharge and urinary incontinence.

Additional procedures intended to give diagnostically useful information are permissible provided they do not interfere with the basic test. For example:
- additional changes and weighing of the collecting device can give information about the timing of urine loss; and
- the collecting device may be an electronic recording pad so that the timing is recorded directly.

## Comment

This type of study is easy to carry out and interpret and provides a great deal of useful information. The weight of urine lost during the test is measured and recorded in grams (g). A loss of less than 1 g is within experimental error and the patient should be regarded as essentially dry.

# FLOW RATE

The simplest and often most useful investigation in the assessment of voiding dysfunction is measurement of a urinary flow rate:
- it is noninvasive;
- it can often be used to confirm the presence of bladder outlet obstruction objectively;
- when combined with measurement of residual urine volume it is an excellent screening test for bladder outlet obstruction in patients who have benign prostatic hyperplasia; and
- it is useful for identifying those patients who require more extensive urodynamic evaluation.

Studies have demonstrated that simple uroflowmetry by itself is adequate investigation for uncomplicated prostate-mediated bladder outflow obstruction in over 60% of patients.

More detailed investigation is indicated in a variety of situations (e.g. where the result which is obtained is at variance with the patient's symptoms or where symptoms remain despite surgical correction).

Measured uroflow is dependent upon a number of factors including:
- detrusor contractility;
- relaxation of the sphincter mechanisms; and
- patency of the urethra.

Flow rate can be normal in the early stages of obstruction due to a compensatory increase in detrusor contractility resulting in a high voiding pressure. This high pressure normal flow voiding (>15 ml/s) occurs in approximately 7–15% of patients with bladder outflow obstruction secondary to BPH. A low flow rate is not diagnostic of bladder outlet obstruction and may be due to obstruction or poor bladder contractility. They can be differentiated by simultaneous measurement of detrusor pressure and flow.

## URODYNAMICS IN PRACTICE: FLOW RATE

- Urinary flow rate is measured with a flowmeter, a device that measures and indicates a quantity of fluid (volume or mass) passed per unit time; such machines usually indicate the volumetric flow rate
- The measurement is expressed in ml/s
- A flow rate estimation can be carried out either by itself or in combination with other techniques
- Patients are instructed to void normally, either sitting or standing, with a comfortably full bladder and should be provided with as much privacy as possible to remove the inhibitory effects of the test environment

**Commonly used flowmeters**
- **Rotating disk method:** the voided fluid is directed onto a rotating disk and the amount landing on the disk produces a proportionate increase in its inertia; the power required to keep the disk rotating at a constant rate is measured, so allowing calculation of the flow rate of fluid
- **Electronic dipstick method:** a dipstick is mounted in a collecting chamber and as urine accumulates the electrical capacitance of the dipstick changes, allowing calculation of the rate of fluid accumulation and hence the flow rate
- **Gravimetric method:** the weight of collected fluid or the hydrostatic pressure at the base of a collecting cylinder is measured. This similarly allows calculation of the flow rate

**Practical points**
The important factors to consider when interpreting a flow rate are:
- volume voided
- rate; and
- pattern (in particular whether the flow is continuous or intermittent).

A number of characteristic traces are shown in Figure 3.3.
Flow rates are dependent upon:
- bladder volume;
- age; and
- sex.

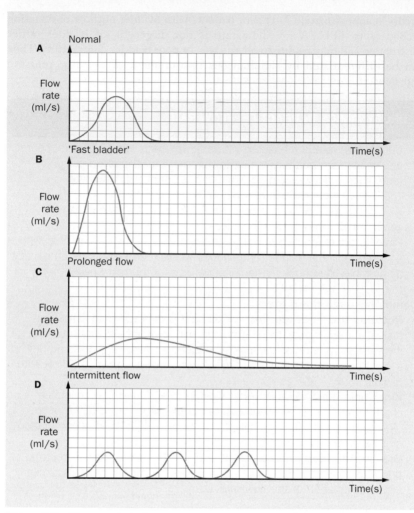

**Figure 3.3 Characteristic flow patterns.** (A) Normal – there is rapid change before and after the peak flow. (B) 'Fast bladder' – an exaggeration of normal associated with high end-filling pressure and seen in cases of detrusor instability. (C) Prolonged flow – associated with relative outflow obstruction. (D) Intermittent flow – resulting from abdominal straining superimposed on poor detrusor function.

When carrying out a urinary flow rate estimation particular attention needs to be paid to the following factors as they can influence the result obtained:

- voided volumes of less than 150 ml can lead to erroneous results and should be repeated, whereas high voided volumes (>600 ml) may

lower flow rates by overstretching the bladder, resulting in detrusor decompensation;
- if possible the patient should be in favourable surroundings and should not be unduly stressed;
- position of the patient when voiding (supine or standing) should be noted;
- whether the flow rate is a so-called 'free flow rate' occurring after natural filling or the bladder is filled using a catheter. The 'free flow rate' is more physiological.

## Comment

The urinary flow rate provides important and useful information about whether there is obstruction to the outflow tract and may indicate a possible aetiology. The normal flow curve is bell-shaped and characterized by a rapid rise to maximal flow where the time to maximum flow does not exceed one-third of the flow time.

Males under 40 years of age generally have maximum urinary flow rates over 25 ml/s. Flow rates decrease with age and men over 60 years of age who do not have urinary obstruction usually have maximum flow rates over 15 ml/s.

Females have higher flow rates than males, usually of the order of 5–10 ml/s more for a given volume. Exaggerated maximum flow rates are typical in women who have genuine stress incontinence, where the outlet resistance is much reduced and in patients who have marked bladder overactivity – the so-called 'fast bladder'.

Patients who have urinary obstruction generally have:
- a low maximum flow rate;
- a prolonged flow time; and
- a slow time to maximum flow.

Patients who have a decompensated detrusor typically demonstrate a straining pattern characterized by an irregular spiking pattern.

Patients who have urethral stricture disease often have a low maximum flow rate, which plateaus in a box-like fashion. A urethral stricture may not cause obstructive voiding symptoms until the urethral calibre is reduced below 11 F.

Uroflowmetry is invaluable in the assessment of voiding function for a wide range of urological conditions. Reliance should be placed on the observed flow pattern as well as any absolute values obtained. The results must always be interpreted within the context of the clinical situation, recognising the limitations of the study.

If there is doubt about the diagnosis after uroflowmetry, more complex urodynamic studies may be required. To provide more detailed information a simple flow rate can be combined with a measurement of the postvoiding residual volume.

**TERMINOLOGY: URINARY FLOW RATE (International Continence Society standardization, 1988; Figure 3.4)**

- **Voided volume:** total volume expelled via the urethra
- **Maximum flow rate (Qmax):** maximum measured flow rate
- **Average flow rate:** voided volume divided by flow time – calculation of average flow rate is only meaningful if flow is continuous and without terminal dribbling
- **Flow time:** time over which measurable flow actually occurs – the flow pattern must be described when flow time and average flow rate are measured
- **Time to maximum flow:** elapsed time from onset of flow to maximum flow
- **Intermittent flow:** the same parameters used to characterize continuous flow can be applicable with care – when measuring flow time the time intervals between flow episodes are disregarded
- **Voiding time:** total duration of micturition (i.e. including interruptions); when voiding is completed without interruption, voiding time is equal to flow time

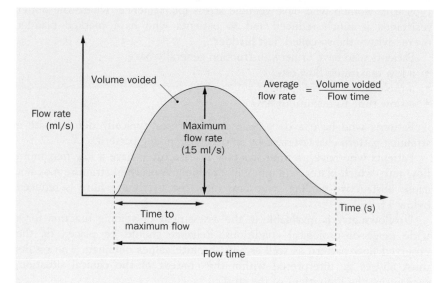

**Figure 3.4  Continuous urine flow recording illustrating the International Continence Society nomenclature.** (Reproduced with permission from Neurourology and Urodynamics 1988; 7:403–426.)

### Artefacts

The flow rate can be misleading. Common artefacts are shown in Figure 3.5 and include:

- straining, which can alter the flow rate and should be taken into account when interpreting results; and
- irregularities in the measured flow rate due to collecting funnel artefacts and variations in direction of the urinary stream.

## ULTRASOUND CYSTODYNAMOGRAM

Ultrasound cystodynamogram (USCD) combines ultrasound with a flow rate measurement to provide more detailed information on bladder function (Figure 3.6). It is a routine investigation for all hospital outpatients who have voiding disorders; an alternative is to measure the residual urine volume by catheterization.

### URODYNAMICS IN PRACTICE: ULTRASOUND CYSTODYNAMOGRAM

- The full bladder is scanned using any form of ultrasound probe allowing adequate visualization of the bladder – patients should be scanned when they feel 'full', so providing an idea of functional bladder capacity
- The patient voids into a flowmeter in private
- A postvoiding scan is taken as soon after voiding as possible to provide accurate assessment of the true bladder residual volume
- Interpretation of the flow rate takes account of the artefacts and factors mentioned in text

### Practical points

Ensure that:

- the patient has a subjectively full bladder before carrying out the study to provide a representative result; and
- the study is carried out in circumstances where the patient can be relaxed to avoid errors.

### Comment

Ultrasound cystodynamograms provide data on:

- bladder capacity;
- flow rate; and
- postvoiding residual volume.
  Their advantages are:
- provision of a more detailed assessment of lower urinary tract function than flow rates alone;

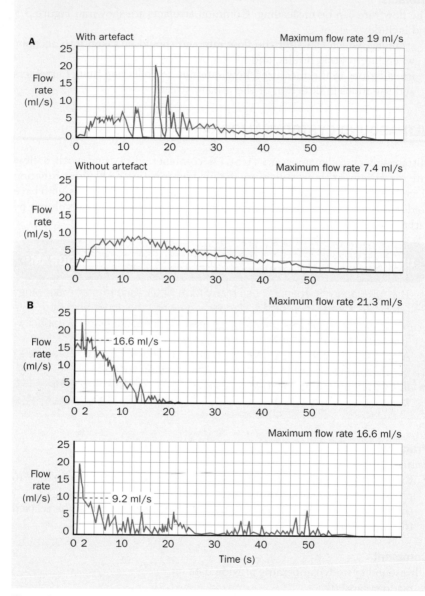

**Figure 3.5 Artefacts.** (A) The artefact (a spurious maximum flow rate of 19 ml/s) results from squeezing the prepuce of the penis during voiding. It is eliminated revealing a true maximum flow rate of 7.4 ml/s when the patient stops squeezing the penis. (B) Both these flow curves show artefactual spikes, but an experienced urologist has corrected the traces (dotted line) so that the true maximum flow rates are 16.6 and 9.2 ml/s, as shown.

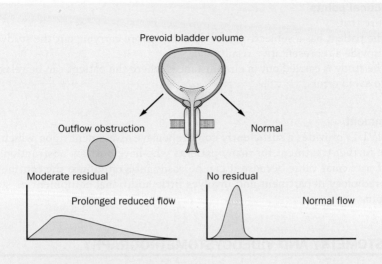

**Figure 3.6  Ultrasound cystodynamogram.**

- easy to do, requiring little specialized equipment;
- noninvasive nature; and
- no need for ionizing radiation.

A USCD is of particular value for following up patients attending clinics (e.g. to follow up a patient who has a hypocontractile detrusor following operative relief of obstruction or for suspected compromised voiding after a repair procedure for stress incontinence).

## INTRAVENOUS URODYNAMOGRAM

The intravenous urodynamogram (IVUD) provides markedly more information than the conventional intravenous urogram (IVU) by virtue of its combination with a free flow rate.

### URODYNAMICS IN PRACTICE: INTRAVENOUS URODYNAMOGRAM

- Provides appropriate upper tract radiographs of an IVU
- Includes a voiding flow rate measured when the patient feels that his or her bladder is naturally full (an event that can be hastened by using a suitable diuretic)
- The subsequent postmicturition film after natural micturition allows accurate assessment of the patient's true bladder residual volume

## Practical points

Ensure that:

- the patient has a subjectively full bladder before carrying out the study to provide a representative result; and
- the study is carried out in circumstances where the patient can be relaxed to avoid errors.

## Comment

An IVUD provides a sufficiently comprehensive assessment upon which to base further treatment for many patients who have outflow obstruction. It is of particular value because it can be easily integrated into the routine of the radiology department and involves little additional equipment or staff training.

# CYSTOMETRY AND VIDEOCYSTOMETROGRAPHY

## Cystometry

Detailed urodynamic investigation is necessary for equivocal or more complex urological cases. Cystometry is the method used to measure the pressure–volume relationships of the bladder. The term cystometry is usually taken to mean measurement of detrusor pressure during controlled bladder filling and subsequent voiding with measurement of the synchronous flow rate (filling and voiding cystometry).

Cystometry helps characterize detrusor function by assessing:

- bladder compliance;
- sensation;
- stability; and
- capacity.

## Simple cystometry

In simple cystometry the intravesical (total bladder) pressure is measured while the bladder is filled. It is not accurate because it assumes that the detrusor pressure approximates to the intravesical pressure. As the bladder is an intra-abdominal organ, the detrusor pressure is subjected to changes in intra-abdominal pressure, which may lead to inaccurate diagnoses.

## Subtracted cystometry

Subtracted cystometry involves measurement of both the intravesical and intra-abdominal pressure simultaneously. Electronic subtraction of the intra-abdominal pressure from the intravesical pressure enables detrusor pressure measurement.

**Videocystometrography** (video = I see; cystometrography = cystometry plus cystourethrography)

If there are appropriate radiological facilities, the bladder can be filled with contrast media to allow simultaneous screening of the bladder and outflow tract during filling and voiding (cystourethrography). Combination of these two procedures results in the gold standard investigation, the videocystometrogram (Figure 3.7).

Radiological screening provides valuable additional anatomical information on:

- the bladder;
- the presence of vesico-ureteral reflux;
- the level of any outflow obstruction in the lower urinary tract; and
- the degree of support to the bladder base during coughing.

By itself radiological screening is more than adequate to make a diagnosis of sphincteric competence. This information, along with the accompanying pressure–flow traces can be recorded on a video tape allowing subsequent review and discussion.

Most patients can be adequately investigated using the simpler urodynamic techniques described earlier in this chapter including simple cystometry. Videocystometry is, however, essential for:

- adequate assessment of complex cases where equivocal results have been obtained from simpler investigations;
- investigation of patients with neuropathic disorders; and
- situations where there has been an apparent failure to respond to a previous operative procedure.

### URODYNAMICS IN PRACTICE: VIDEOCYSTOMETROGRAPHY AND CYSTOMETRY (Figure 3.8)

- Detrusor pressure is estimated by the automatic subtraction of rectal pressure (as an index of intra-abdominal pressure) from the total bladder pressure (intravesical pressure), so removing the influence of artefacts produced by abdominal straining
- During the study, notes are made of initial bladder residual volume, bladder volume at the time of the patient's first sensation of filling, final tolerated bladder volume, and final residual volume after voiding
- All systems are zeroed at atmospheric pressure – for external transducers the reference point is the level of the superior edge of the symphysis pubis; for a catheter-mounted transducer the reference point is the transducer itself
- Patients, excluding those who have indwelling catheters, are asked to void into a flowmeter to allow measurement of a free flow rate
- They are then requested to lie in the left lateral position on an X-ray screening table while a 2 mm diameter saline-filled catheter is

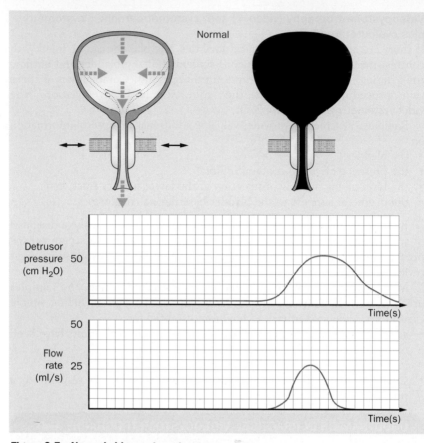

**Figure 3.7** **Normal videocystometrogram.**

introduced into the rectum, the end of the tube being protected with a finger stall to prevent faecal blockage (a slit is cut in this to prevent tamponade producing artefactual results during the study)
- With patients in the supine position, the external urethral meatus is cleaned with antiseptic solution
- The urethra in males is anaesthetized with 1% lignocaine gel containing chlorhexidine
- A 10 F Nelaton filling catheter with a 1 mm diameter saline-filled plastic pressure catheter inserted into the subterminal site hole is gently inserted into the bladder and the two catheters are then disengaged
- The bladder is filled via the 10 F catheter, which is removed before the voiding phase leaving the fine catheter *in situ*

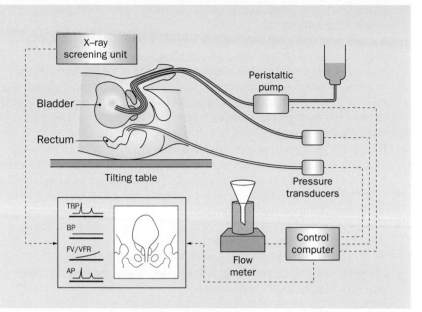

**Figure 3.8 Schematic diagram of videocystometrography and videocystometry.**
The bladder is filled at a predetermined rate with a radio-opaque contrast medium with the simultaneous measurement of bladder pressure (TBP) and rectal pressure (AP). The true detrusor pressure (BP) is calculated automatically (TBP–AP). Infused volume (FV) and the voiding flow rate (VFR) are recorded. This information with accompanying radiographic pictures and a sound track is recorded on video tape allowing subsequent review and analysis.

- Alternatively a 6–8 F biluminal catheter can be used, which avoids the need to use two catheters and then disengage them
- The bladder is drained of urine and this initial residual volume is recorded
- Alternatively the study can be carried out by filling on top of the initial residual volume and calculating the residual at the end of the study by subtraction
- The two pressure measurement lines are connected to the transducers incorporated in the urodynamic apparatus
- The lines are flushed through with saline, great care being taken to exclude all air bubbles from both the tubing and transducer chambers
- Contrast medium or saline (in a nonvideo study) at room temperature is then instilled into the bladder at a predetermined rate under the control of a peristaltic pump – medium and fast fill (50–100 ml/min) is used routinely in our unit, but slower filling rates (10–20 ml/min)

approaching the physiological range are mandatory when assessing a neuropathic bladder

- It is our practice to fill the bladder initially in the supine position and note the volume at first sensation of filling – when the patient first experiences discomfort, the radiographic table is tipped towards the standing position and subsequent bladder filling is discontinued at the maximum tolerated capacity; during bladder filling the patient is asked to consciously suppress bladder contraction and may be asked to cough or heel bounce
- The patient is then turned to the oblique position relative to the X-ray machine and is asked to cough to demonstrate if sphincteric weakness is present and is then asked to void into the flowmeter provided
- In units where a tipping table is not available the study can be carried out in the sitting or standing position initially
- Stand the patient upright at the end of the study to assess whether there is postural detrusor instability
- In the absence of radiological screening stress incontinence is assessed with the patient lying flat with legs abducted and standing with legs slightly apart, and squatting
- Throughout the study continuous rectal pressure, total bladder pressure, and electronically subtracted detrusor pressure (total bladder pressure minus rectal pressure) measurements are sampled at a predetermined rate (usually 1 Hz) and the results displayed on the video display unit or stored to disc or polygraph chart recorder depending upon the equipment in use
- Quality control is obtained by asking the patient to cough at regular intervals (Figure 3.9)

## Cystometry or videocystometrography?

Most urodynamic units do not have the benefit of combined fluoroscopic screening with urodynamics or video recording facilities. Although it is advantageous to be able to perform such tests within a radiography department on a temporary or permanent basis, simple cystometry may suffice in the routine assessment of patients presenting with urinary frequency and urgency. Similarly, stress incontinence without urinary frequency or urgency does not necessarily require investigation by urodynamics and if stress incontinence is not clinically demonstrable, cystography alone may be all that is required to demonstrate the anatomical situation before operative correction.

Synchronous cystography and cystometry recordings (videocysto-metrography, VCMG) are most important in the assessment of complex urological cases, particularly if there has been a failure to respond to a previous operation because this investigation allows a combined anatomical and functional evaluation of lower urinary tract function. Nevertheless simple

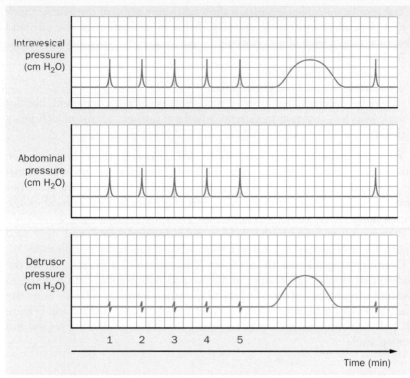

**Figure 3.9  Quality control during urodynamics.** The patient is asked to cough every 1 minute before, during and after the test.

cystourethrography can be carried out in all radiography departments. A cough test during cystography may be all that is required to confirm a diagnosis of simple stress incontinence not accompanied by urinary frequency or urgency that cannot be demonstrated clinically before operative correction.

## Videourodynamics
### Evaluation of female incontinence
Videodynamics is an excellent method for evaluating the urethral outlet in female patients who have urinary incontinence. Standing quietly and partially obliqued, the bladder neck position may be abnormally low, below the level of the upper third of the symphysis pubis, signifying loss of pelvic floor support in patients who have hypermobile urethras or anatomical stress incontinence. Coughing or Valsalva manoeuvres cause these vesicourethral units to descend and leak. On termination of the increased intra-abdominal pressure the bladder neck quickly 'springs back' to its original position terminating leakage.

The semilateral/oblique position allows differentiation of the bladder neck from a dependent cystocoele and also helps in evaluation of the size and functional significance of a cystocoele.

Beaking of the bladder neck:

- is probably a normal finding;
- is common in continent females; but
- should be differentiated from a rectangular-shaped incompetent bladder neck, which is common in patients who have intrinsic sphincter deficiency (ISD).

Typically patients who have pure ISD causing their incontinence demonstrate severe leakage with minimal increases in intra-abdominal pressure and minimal urethrovesical hypermobility. The urethra does not spring back, but appears to stay open and continues leaking even after the stress event.

Patients often have both bladder neck hypermobility and ISD and experience is necessary to interpret their relative functional significance.

Cystourethrography via the adjacent X-ray screening apparatus allows the synchronous display of pressure and flow and radiographic data relating to bladder morphology (e.g. diverticula, vesicoureteral reflux, and the appearances of the bladder outlet and urethra) on a video display unit (Figure 3.10). The monitor images can be recorded on video tape allowing review and detailed study.

### General comments

The residual urine may be measured before starting to fill the bladder. However, the removal of a large volume of residual urine may alter detrusor function, especially in neuropathic disorders. Similarly, cystometeric parameters may be markedly changed by rapid filling rates in neurogenic patients. In both instances, the measured maximum cystometric capacity and bladder compliance may be falsely lowered.

During cystometry it is taken for granted that the patient is awake, unanaesthetized, and neither sedated nor taking drugs that affect bladder function. Any variations from this ideal must be taken into account when interpreting results.

In a substantial number of women who present with incontinence, urinary leakage cannot be demonstrated either clinically or radiologically; monitoring by assessing the amount of leakage into pads can be particularly helpful in this situation. Similarly, continuous ambulatory urodynamic monitoring is invaluable for a small group of patients who have marked symptoms, but with no demonstrable urodynamic abnormality on conventional testing.

The bladder neck mechanism fails to relax during voiding in a small percentage of young men resulting in the clinical entity of bladder neck

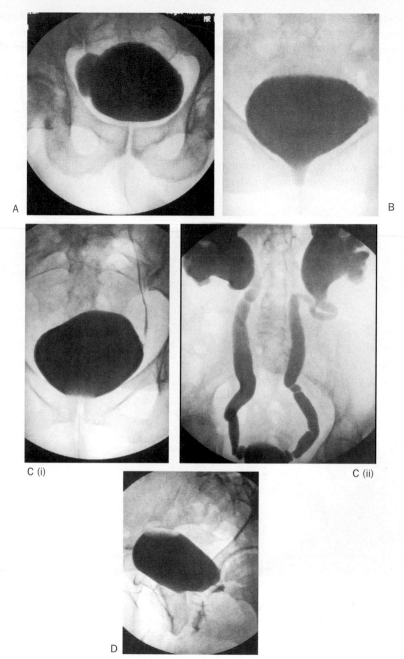

**Figure 3.10 Videocystourethrograms.** (A) Diverticulum. (B) Small diverticulum and stress incontinence. (C) Reflux: (i) mild left reflux; (ii) marked bilateral reflux. (D) Vesicovaginal fistula.

obstruction (dyssynergia). This abnormality is evident during videocystometry if the patient is asked to inhibit micturition voluntarily. In a normal urodynamic study contrast media will be milked back from the distal sphincter mechanism proximally through the bladder neck into the bladder – a normal stop test. If there is obstruction at the level of the bladder neck contrast will be trapped within the prostatic urethra (Figure 3.11).

## Practical points

A number of variations in technique are currently available and the following aspects deserve specific consideration.

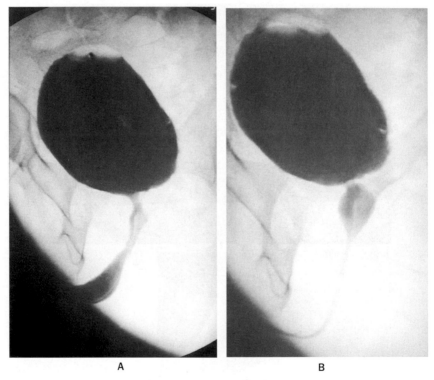

A                                               B

**Figure 3.11   Detrusor–bladder neck dyssynergia.** During a urodynamic study if the patient is asked to inhibit micturition voluntarily, contrast medium will be milked back from the distal sphincter mechanism proximally through the bladder neck into the bladder. If there is obstruction at the level of the bladder neck, contrast will be trapped within the prostatic urethra. (A) Voiding study in a patient with bladder neck obstruction. (B) Voluntary inhibition of voiding in this patient illustrating 'trapping' of contrast.

### Access

Most cystometry is carried out using the transurethral route, but in paediatric patients the urodynamics catheter is sometimes placed percutaneously in a suprapubic position (usually under a previous anaesthetic) for both bladder filling and pressure measurement.

### Type of catheter

Considerations include:

- for fluid-filled catheters – specify the number of catheters, whether they have single or multiple lumens, type, and size. Catheters larger than or equal to 8 F may introduce obstruction artefact and should not be utilized.
- for catheter tip transducers – the specifications vary between manufacturers; the catheters tend to be expensive and too fragile for routine use.

### Measuring equipment

Many commercial urodynamic systems are currently available and they vary greatly in terms of sampling rate, associated computer software backup, and price.

A major problem with existing computer programs is the ease with which they will record artefacts, which can then bias the results of the subsequent automatic data analysis. Investigators are advised to maintain a real time paper output from their computer program wherever possible to allow cross-checking for artefacts. Investigators are also strongly advised not to rely upon the computer-generated data sheets, but to use an appropriate proforma that allows interpretation of the urodynamic findings by the investigator (Figure 3.12).

### Test medium (liquid or gas)

The advantage of equipment using gas as a medium is that it can be more compact and is therefore more easily portable. A major drawback with gas cystometry – aerodynamics! – is its susceptibility to artefact resulting from changes in the temperature of the gaseous medium (a much less important consideration when fluid is used). Fluid cystometry (sterile water, normal saline or contrast) is the medium of choice in the majority of cases. It is recommended to maintain the fluid at room temperature recognizing that colder fluids can precipitate bladder instability.

### Position of patient

The patient's position (i.e. supine, sitting, or standing) must be considered.

### Type of filling

Bladder filling may be by diuresis or catheter. Filling by catheter may be continuous or incremental and the precise filling rate should be stated. When

**43**

## Conventional urodynamic report

*Patient Details:*  *Date of study:*  /  /

| | | 1 | **Fill Number** | 2 |
|---|---|---|---|---|

**Filling** Fill rate (ml/min) ☐☐☐  ☐☐☐
Baseline Pdet (cmH$_2$O) ☐☐☐  ☐☐☐
First sensation filling (ml)* ☐☐☐  ☐☐☐
Cystometric capacity (ml)* ☐☐☐  ☐☐☐
Compliance (0=normal; 1=reduced) ☐  ☐
**Instability**
Fill (0=nil; 1=systolic; 2=nonsystolic) ☐  ☐
Cough ☐  ☐
Posture ☐  ☐

| Contraction no. | 1 | 2 | 3 | 4 | 5 | 1 | 2 | 3 | 4 | 5 |
|---|---|---|---|---|---|---|---|---|---|---|
| Vol. at contraction | | | | | | | | | | |
| Max. rise in Pdet | | | | | | | | | | |

End-filling Pdet (cmH$_2$O) ☐☐☐  ☐☐☐

*Filling volume (need to add initial residual in formal data recording)

**Voiding** Opening Pdet (cmH$_2$O) ☐☐☐  ☐☐☐
Pdet.max (cmH$_2$O) (Not Pdet.iso) ☐☐☐  ☐☐☐
Pdet at peak flow (ml/s) ☐☐☐  ☐☐☐
Peak flow rate (ml/s) ☐☐.☐  ☐☐.☐
Pdet.iso (cmH$_2$O) ☐☐☐  ☐☐☐
After contraction (0=no; 1=yes) ☐  ☐
Pdet (cmH$_2$O) ☐☐☐  ☐☐☐
Volume voided (ml) ☐☐☐  ☐☐☐
Residual urine (ml) ☐☐☐  ☐☐☐
Calculated initial residual urine (ml) ☐☐☐  ☐☐☐

 R  L

**Video** Bladder outline ☐  VUR Grade ☐  ☐
1=normal; 2=trabeculated;  Grade as defined by International Reflux Study Group (Grades 1–5)
3=sacculated; 4=multiple diverticula

 Males  Females
Bladder neck ☐  ☐
In men: 1=normal opening with void; 2=poor opening
In women: 1=closed; 2=open with fill;
3=open with standing; 4=open with stress

Stop test (M)/Position (F) ☐  ☐
In men: 1=normal; 2=trapping present; 3=equivocal; 9=not done
In women: 4=well supported; 5=descent on stress; 6=prolapse

Prostatic urethra ☐ 1=normal opening; 2=attenuated;
3=DSD; 4=indeterminate

Anterior urethra ☐ 1=normal; 2=stricture; 3=unsure

**Comments/Report**

**Figure 3.12 Proforma for interpreting urodynamic findings.** (DSD, detrusor–sphincter dyssynergia; Pdet, detrusor pressure; VUR, vesicoureteral reflux.)

an incremental method is used the volume increment should be stated. Asking patients to change position from supine to standing is a commonly performed provocative manoeuvre for bladder instability. Many patients will only demonstrate stress urinary incontinence when standing. Immobile patients (e.g. spinal-cord-injured patients) are usually studied supine and rotated to the lateral oblique position.

### Continuous or intermittent pressure measurement
Although continuous pressure measurement is of greatest use in clinical practice (e.g. in patients who have a suprapubic catheter in place and where a urethral pressure line cannot be introduced through the urethra), alternate incremental filling of the bladder with staged measurement of the pressures can be carried out using the same catheter.

### Who carries out the study and how? – data quality
It is essential that urodynamic studies are carried out or supervised by experienced investigators and important aspects are:
- always take a clinical history from the patient at the time of carrying out the study and counsel the patient before attending on the day and at the start of the study about the nature of the test;
- make sure that the machinery is regularly serviced and calibrate the transducers on a regular basis;
- make sure that the lines are zeroed at the start of the study and check that subtraction is perfect before starting the study and every minute during the study by asking the patient to cough – if in doubt about artefact repeat the study;
- choose the correct filling rate for the study (e.g. slow filling at a rate of 10–20 ml/s for patients who have a neuropathic bladder and those who have a reduced functional capacity).

### Normal values
During cystometry, under normal circumstances the bladder should fill to a capacity of approximately 500 ml before there is a strong desire to void (and often less in women as compared to men). During subsequent bladder filling whilst the patient is making a conscious effort to inhibit voiding, the subtracted intravesical detrusor pressure should not increase much from its baseline value. It is recommended that the bladder should not be overfilled in patients with large capacities, above 650–700 ml, as little additional information is obtained.

The International Continence Society no longer recognises a specific value as essential for the diagnosis of detrusor instability, and in contemporary practice it can be said to be present if there is a physiological pressure rise off the baseline. The only exception is represented by a gradual linear rise in pressure during detrusor filling – so-called low compliance, which is clearly defined (see below), but remains an as yet poorly classified entity.

During subsequent voiding the patient's bladder empties completely with a maximum detrusor pressure of 25–50 cm $H_2O$ and maximum urinary flow rates of over 25 ml/s in men under 40 years and over 15 ml/s in men over 60 years and over 30–35 ml/s in women.

## Compliance

Compliance indicates the change in volume for a given change in pressure. It is calculated by dividing the volume change ($\delta V$) by the change in detrusor pressure ($\delta Pdet$) during the change in bladder volume. $C = \delta V / \delta Pdet$. Compliance is expressed as ml/cm $H_2O$.

### TERMINOLOGY: CYSTOMETRY (International Continence Society standardization, 1988) (Figure 3.13)

**Filling rates**
- **Slow fill:** <10 ml/min) – a 'physiological' filling
- **Medium fill:** 10–100 ml/min
- **Rapid fill:** >100 ml/min

**Bladder pressure measurements during filling**
- **Intravesical pressure:** the pressure within the bladder
- **Abdominal pressure:** the pressure surrounding the bladder, which is estimated from rectal or, less commonly, extraperitoneal pressure – the simultaneous measurement of abdominal pressure is essential for interpreting the intravesical pressure trace; however, artefacts on the detrusor pressure trace may be produced by intrinsic rectal contractions
- **Detrusor pressure:** the component of intravesical pressure created by forces in the bladder wall (passive and active) and estimated by subtracting abdominal pressure from intravesical pressure

**Bladder sensation**
- Difficult to evaluate because of its subjective nature – usually assessed by questioning the patient about his or her sensation of the fullness of the bladder during cystometry
- **First desire to void**
- **Normal desire to void:** the feeling that leads the patient to pass urine at the next convenient moment, but voiding can be delayed if necessary
- **Strong desire to void:** a persistent desire to void without the fear of leakage
- **Urgency:** a strong desire to void accompanied by fear of leakage or fear of pain

- **Pain:** the site and character should be specified; pain during bladder filling or micturition is abnormal

**Capacity**
- The term capacity must be qualified
- **Maximum cystometric capacity:** the volume at which a patient who has normal sensation feels that he or she can no longer delay micturition; it cannot be defined in the same terms in the absence of sensation and is then the volume at which the clinician decides to terminate filling; it may be markedly increased in the presence of sphincter incompetence by occlusion of the urethra (e.g. by a Foley catheter)
- **Functional bladder capacity or voided volume:** more relevant than maximum cystometric capacity and is assessed from a volume–frequency chart (urinary diary).
- **Maximum (anaesthetic) bladder capacity:** the volume measured after filling during a deep general, spinal or epidural anaesthetic, specifying fluid temperature, filling pressure, and filling time

## Assessing leakage and testing for sphincteric insufficiency
### Detrusor leak point pressure
This is the subtracted or detrusor pressure at which leakage occurs. It measures the capacity of the bladder neck and urethral sphincter mechanism to resist increases in intraabdominal pressure. It is a term used when assessing patients who have neuropathic disorders and a closed or spastic outlet. In the group of patients who have a high filling pressure 'closed system' the upper tracts have an increased risk of being damaged if there is a subtracted detrusor pressure pressure of more than 30–40 cm $H_2O$ documented during filling cystometry. It is important to realize that neurogenic patients can have dangerously high detrusor leak point pressures even though they have stress urinary incontinence and low abdominal leak points secondary to intrinsic sphincter deficiency.

### Abdominal leak point pressure
This is the abdominal pressure at which leakage occurs and acts as a crude measure of the ability of the bladder neck and urethral sphincter mechanism to resist increases in intraabdominal pressure. Its measurement poses a major problem for comparing results because there is no standard technique with regard to:
- threshold values (not defined);
- catheter calibre;
- presence of prolapse;
- bladder volume;
- Valsalva manoeuvre versus cough;

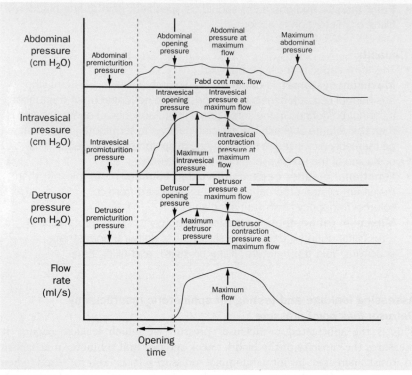

**Figure 3.13 Pressure–flow recordings of micturition with International Continence Society nomenclature.** (Reproduced with permission from the Scandinavian Journal of Urology and Nephrology, 1988; 114.)

- straining (contraction and relaxation of the pelvic floor); and
- measurement baseline.

It is generally accepted that patients with anatomic stress incontinence typically have high abominal leak point pressures >100 cm $H_2O$ while patients with ISD leak with pressures <60 cm $H_2O$. It is important to point out that the abdominal leak point pressure by itself is not diagnostic of intrinsic sphincter deficiency and should be correlated with other clinical parameters.

There are many contradictory reports on the correlation between urethral pressure and leak point pressure. Our experience would support the use of graduated coughs to assess leakage, ideally coupled with cystourethrography and videocystometry.

**TERMINOLOGY: BLADDER PRESSURE MEASUREMENTS DURING MICTURITION (see Figure 3.13)**

(The specifications of patient position, access for pressure measurement, catheter type, and measuring equipment are as for cystometry.)

- **Opening time:** time elapsing from the initial rise in detrusor pressure to onset of flow; it is the initial isovolumetric contraction period of micturition; time lags should be taken into account – in most urodynamic systems there is a time lag equal to the time taken for the urine to pass from the point of pressure measurement to the uroflow transducer

**Intravesical, abdominal, and detrusor pressure curves**
- **Premicturition pressure:** pressure recorded immediately before the initial isovolumetric contraction
- **Opening pressure:** pressure recorded at the onset of measured flow
- **Maximum pressure:** maximum value of measured pressure
- **Pressure at maximum flow:** pressure at maximum measured flow rate
- **Contraction pressure at maximum flow:** difference between pressure at maximum flow and premicturition pressure
- **Postmicturition events (e.g. after contractions):** these are not well understood and cannot yet be defined (Figure 3.20)

**Pressure–flow relationships**

In the past the flow rate and voiding pressure were related as a 'urethral resistance factor'. The concept of a resistance factor originated from rigid tube hydrodynamics. However, the urethra does not generally behave as a rigid tube because it is an irregular and distensible conduit with walls and surroundings that have active and passive elements that influence the flow through it. Therefore a resistance factor cannot provide a valid comparison between patients.

There are many ways of displaying the relationships between flow and pressure during micturition. As yet, available data do not permit a standard presentation of pressure–flow parameters.

Contemporary views over the display of the pressure–flow relationship have proved to be contentious and there is a variety of suggested mathematical models. The comparison of these is best achieved by referrring to the latest World Health Organization consultation on BPH (Figures 3.14a-f).

The results of pressure-flow studies can be classified according to a number of nomograms, the most popular being the Abrams–Griffiths nomogram and the Schafer linear passive urethral resistance relation (LinPURR). Patients are conveniently classified as obstructed, unobstructed and equivocally obstructed

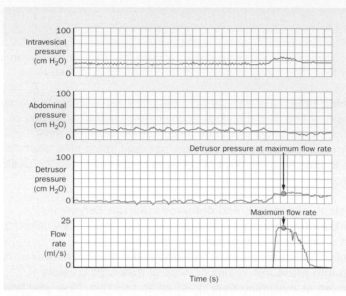

**Figure 3.14a   Typical pressure–flow study obtained when there is no obstruction.** (Reproduced with permission from WHO 4th International Consultation on BPH.)

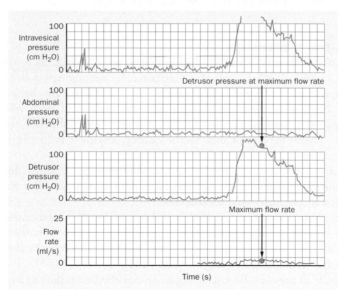

**Figure 3.14b   Pressure–flow study in bladder obstruction.** There is a low maximum flow rate and a maximum detrusor pressure of more than 100 cm $H_2O$. (Reproduced with permission from WHO 4th International Consultation on BPH.)

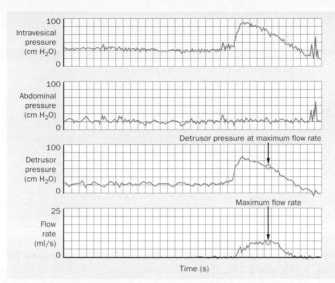

**Figure 3.14c   Pressure–flow study with intermediate (equivocal) values for maximum flow rate and detrusor pressure.** Small rectal contractions are visible in the abdominal pressure trace and are therefore also seen in the detrusor pressure trace as downward deflections. (Reproduced with permission from WHO 4th International Consultation on BPH.)

utilizing the Abrams–Griffiths nomogram (Figure 3.14d). The LinPURR grades detrusor contractility on a scale from very weak (VW) to strong (ST) and quantifies obstruction from grade 0 (no obstruction) to 6 (severe obstruction) (Figure 3.14e). A number of other suggested mathematical models exist, and the comparison of these is best achieved by referring to the latest World Health Organization consultation on BPH (Figure 3.14f). Though the Abrams–Griffiths nomogram is more commonly used because of its simplicity none of these models is routinely used in clinical practice.

There is a high concordance between the various models (Figure 3.15), which has led to the development of the International Continence Society provisional nomogram (Figure 3.16). An individual pressure–flow study can be easily classified by calculating the Abrams–Griffiths number, which is obtained by subtracting twice the maximum flow rate in ml/s from the detrusor pressure at maximum flow in cm $H_2O$. $AG = PdetQmax - 2Qmax$. Obstruction is present if the number is more than 40 with the equivocal zone lying between 20 and 40, and unobstructed being <20 cm $H_2O$.

### Residual urine
Residual urine is the volume of fluid remaining in the bladder immediately following the completion of micturition. Its measurement forms an integral

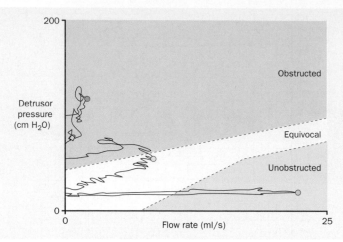

**Figure 3.14d Pressure–flow plots using the Abrams–Griffiths nomogram for Figures 3.14a, 3.14b, and 3.14c.** The maximum flow rates for each trace (representing the pressure–flow data for the whole of each void from Figures 3.14a, 3.14b, and 3.14c) are indicated by coloured dots. For the simpler methods of analysing pressure–flow data, only the location of these dots is important (i.e. in the obstructed, equivocal or nonobstructed region of the nomogram). (Reproduced with permission from WHO 4th International Consultation on BPH.)

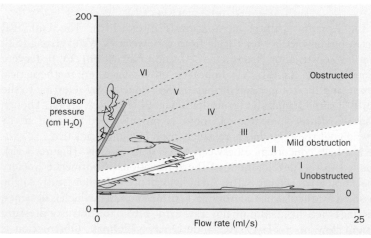

**Figure 3.14e Pressure–flow plots using the LinPURR method for Figures 3.14a, 3.14b, and 3.14c.** The lower part of each plot is approximated by a straight line. The location of the highest end of the line is the maximum flow point and determines the LinPURR grade, ranging from 0–VI, which correlates with different grades of obstruction as indicated. (The LinPURR method of clarifying obstruction was developed by Schafer W. Neurourology and Urodynamics 1985; 4:161–201. Reproduced with permission from WHO 4th International Consultation on BPH.)

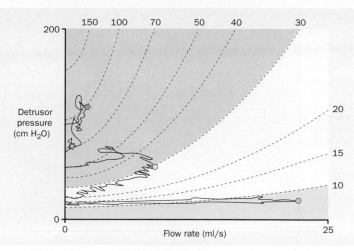

**Figure 3.14f   Pressure–flow plots using the URA method for Figures 3.14a, 3.14b, and 3.14c.** The urethral resistance (URA) was based on analysis of traces from 193 patients and subsequently modified. (Rollema & Van Mastrigt. Journal of Urology 1992; 148:111–116. Reproduced with permission from WHO 4th International Consultation on BPH.)

part of the study of micturition. However, voiding in unfamiliar surroundings can produce unrepresentative results, as may voiding on command with a partially filled or overfilled bladder.

A number of the urodynamic studies discussed earlier in this chapter measure the bladder residual volume. For each individual patient it is necessary to choose a method that is appropriate for the overall assessment of the clinical problem.

Important factors in the interpretation of residual volume include:
- measurement of voided volume and the time interval between voiding and residual urine estimation – this is particularly important if the patient is in a diuretic phase;
- re-entry of urine into the bladder after micturition if there is vesicoureteral reflux – may be falsely interpreted as residual urine;
- urine in bladder diverticula following micturition – a diverticulum can be regarded as either part of the bladder cavity or outside the functioning bladder;
- absence of residual urine – usually a clinically useful observation, but does not exclude intravesical obstruction or bladder dysfunction; and
- isolated finding of residual urine – requires confirmation before being considered significant.

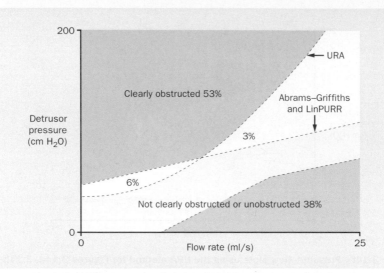

**Figure 3.15  Comparison of the mathematical models for pressure–flow relationships.** There is high concordance between the areas of the pressure–flow plot in which the International Continence Society provisional nomogram, the Abrams–Griffiths nomogram, the LinPURR and the URA agree in identifying obstruction. (Reproduced with permission from WHO 4th International Consultation on BPH.)

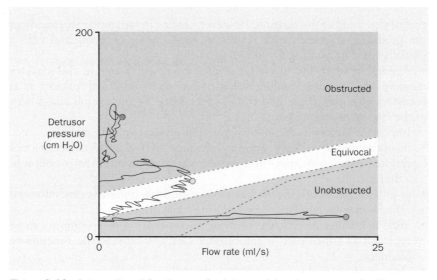

**Figure 3.16  International Continence Society provisional nomogram for Figures 3.14a, 3.14b, and 3.14c.**

## Troubleshooting pressure–flow urodynamics

Many clinical scenarios can be a source of confusion and lead to errors in the interpretation of results.

### Poor subtraction

The rectal and bladder lines are not functioning properly (Figure 3.17). It is remedied by asking the patient to cough at the start of the study and every minute during the study to check the subtraction (Figure 3.9). If cough transmission on one or other line appears inadequate, flush out the lines to clear out air bubbles. As a last resort replace the measurement catheter and if no better suspect a transducer error (rare).

### Negative rectal pressure

A negative rectal pressure adds to the total bladder pressure, and therefore the subtracted bladder pressure (detrusor pressure) may be higher than the

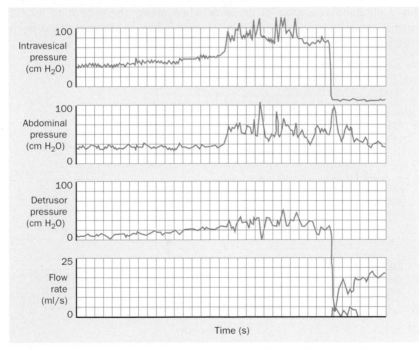

Time (s)

**Figure 3.17  An example of a pressure-flow study that is uninterpretable because of an artefact.** Even prior to the catheter measuring intravesical pressure being ejected at the start of voiding, there is a period when the patient may be straining. During this period the intravesical pressure line appears to be malfunctioning, resulting in inadequate subtraction. (Reproduced with permission from WHO 4th International Consultation on BPH.)

total bladder pressure (Figure 3.18). It is prevented by calibrating the lines adequately at the start of the study and avoiding air bubbles; place a finger cot around the rectal line to prevent blockage of the line by faeculent material and cut a slit in it to prevent tamponade when flushing out the line.

### Cough or giggle instability
This uncommon but well-documented abnormality can be an important cause of symptoms in women (Figure 3.19).

### After contraction
This potential cause of confusion is not well understood and its true significance remains unclear (Figure 3.20).

### Isometric pressure contraction (piso)
This is obtained as a spike of pressure when asking the patient to inhibit micturition and perform a 'stop test' (Figure 3.21). In the past it has been

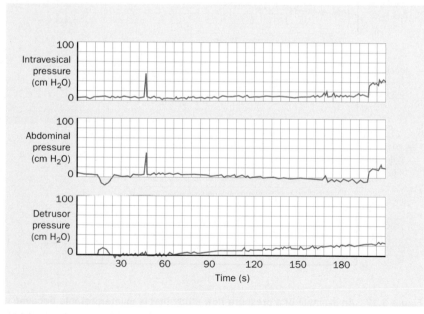

**Figure 3.18 Pressure–flow traces obtained when a negative rectal pressure adds to the total bladder pressure.** The resulting subtracted bladder pressure (detrusor pressure) is higher than the total bladder pressure.

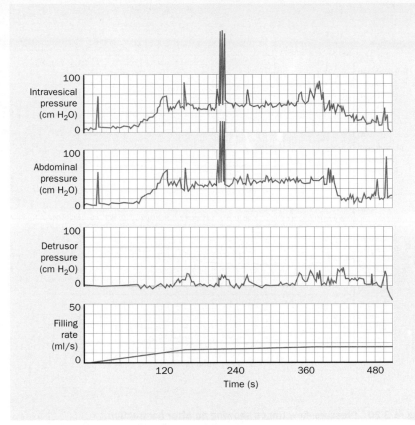

**Figure 3.19    Pressure–flow traces showing cough or giggle instability.**

said to be a sign of detrusor 'power'. This is not particularly useful or of diagnostic value.

## COMPLEX URODYNAMIC INVESTIGATION

The current techniques available for the investigation of urethral sphincteric dysfunction are far from satisfactory:

- urethral pressure profilometry is useful for assessing the effects of sympatholytic agents in drug trials, but is not appropriate as a diagnostic technique;

**57**

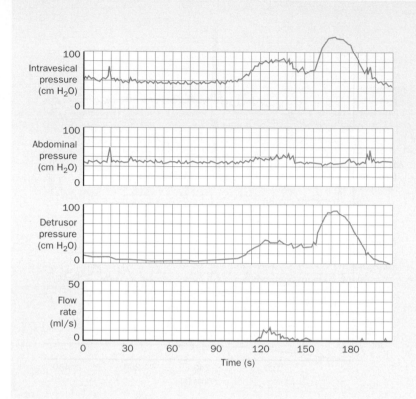

**Figure 3.20   Pressure–flow traces showing an after contraction.**

- dynamic evaluation of urethral sphincter function using anal- or skin-mounted electrodes is inaccurate; and
- accurate electromyographic evaluation of the urethral sphincter is possible with a concentric needle electrode, but is a painful investigation and cannot be carried out during voiding without influencing voiding.

## URETHRAL PRESSURE MEASUREMENT

At rest the urethra is closed and this must be considered when interpreting the results of urethral pressure studies. The urethral pressure and urethral closure pressure are therefore idealized concepts that represent the ability of

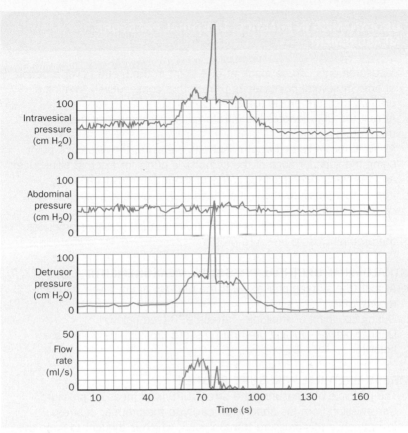

**Figure 3.21    Pressure flow traces obtained showing an isometric pressure contraction.**

the urethra to prevent leakage. In current urodynamic practice the urethral pressure is measured by a number of techniques, which do not always yield consistent values. Not only do the values differ with the method of measurement, but there is often lack of consistency for a single method; for example:

- the effect of catheter rotation when urethral pressure is measured by a catheter-mounted transducer; and
- the considerable artefacts that automatically result from the introduction of any catheter into the urethra.

## URODYNAMICS IN PRACTICE: URETHRAL PRESSURE MEASUREMENT

- Measurements can be made at one point in the urethra over a period of time or several points along the urethra consecutively forming a urethral pressure profile (UPP)
- At rest the UPP denotes the intraluminal pressure along the length of the urethra
- All systems are zeroed at atmospheric pressure, the reference point being the superior edge of the symphysis pubis for external transducers and the transducer itself for catheter-mounted transducers
- Intravesical pressure should be measured to exclude a simultaneous detrusor contraction
- Subtraction of intravesical pressure from urethral pressure produces the urethral closure pressure profile

### INTRALUMINAL URETHRAL PRESSURE MEASUREMENTS
- At rest (the storage phase), with the bladder at any given volume – resting UPP
- During coughing or straining – stress UPP (see below)
- During voiding – voiding urethral pressure profilometry (VUPP, see below)

### STRESS URETHRAL PRESSURE PROFILE
- The principle of measuring the stress UPP is to measure pressure transmission from the abdominal cavity to the urethra; in stress incontinence this pressure transmission, which is thought to keep the normal urethra closed during stress, is inadequate – the urethral closure pressure becomes negative on coughing (Figure 3.24)

#### Fluid bridge test
- A related but different test of bladder neck competence relies upon the continuity of fluid between the bladder and urethra when there is bladder neck incompetence – pressure transmission is measured down the infusion channel of a standard Brown–Wickham perfusion catheter (see below) but with the perfusion switched off

### VOIDING URETHRAL PRESSURE PROFILOMETRY (VUPP)
- Used to determine the pressure and site of urethral obstruction
- Pressure is recorded in the urethra during voiding
- Technique is similar to that used for UPP measured during storage
- Accurate interpretation depends upon simultaneous measurement of intravesical pressure and measurement of pressure at a precisely

localized point in the urethra – localization may be achieved by a radio-opaque marker on the catheter allowing the pressure measurements to be related to a visualized point in the urethra

## URETHRAL PRESSURE PROFILOMETRY
- Three principal techniques currently available – the perfusion method, catheter-mounted transducers, and balloon catheter profilometry – which ever is used it is essential to use a sufficiently sensitive recording apparatus

### Perfusion method
- The perfusion method first described by Brown and Wickham (Figure 3.22) is most widely used
- The catheter has a dual lumen – one for pressure measurements opening at the end of the catheter and the other for perfusion via two opposing side holes 5 cm from the tip of the catheter
- The catheter is constantly perfused at a set rate using a syringe pump (2–10 ml/min) while being withdrawn at a speed of less than 0.7 ml/s

### Catheter-mounted transducers
- These eliminate errors associated with the use of fluid (leaks and air bubbles), but introduce artefacts related to the orientation of the catheter-mounted transducers

### Balloon catheter profilometry
- Uses a small soft balloon mounted on a catheter
- Pressure is transmitted by a fluid column to the external pressure transducer
- Measures urethral pressure accurately, but this catheter is more difficult to use than the catheters used for the other two methods described above

### Practical points
Simultaneous recording of both intravesical and intraurethral pressures is essential during urethral profilometry.

The following information is essential when interpreting the results of such studies:
- infusion medium (liquid or gas);
- rate of infusion;
- stationary, continuous, or intermittent withdrawal;
- rate of withdrawal;
- bladder volume; and
- position of patient (supine, sitting, or standing).

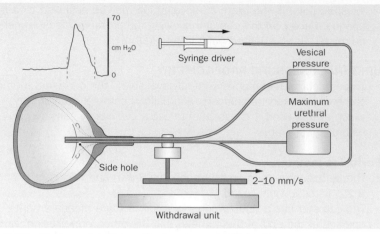

**Figure 3.22  Diagram showing urethral pressure profilometry.**

## TERMINOLOGY: URETHRAL PRESSURE PROFILES (Figure 3.23)

- **Maximum urethral pressure:** maximum pressure of the measured profile
- **Maximum urethral closure pressure:** maximum difference between the urethral pressure and the intravesical pressure
- **Functional profile length:** length of the urethra along which the urethral pressure exceeds intravesical pressure
- **Functional profile length (on stress):** length over which the urethral pressure exceeds the intravesical pressure on stress
- **Pressure 'transmission' ratio:** the increment in urethral pressure on stress as a percentage of the simultaneously recorded increment in intravesical pressure (Figure 3.24); it can be obtained at any point along the urethra for stress profiles obtained during coughing; if a single value is given, the position in the urethra should be stated; if several pressure transmission ratios are defined at different points along the urethra, a pressure 'transmission' profile is obtained; during 'cough profiles' the amplitude of the cough should be stated if possible as measured from the intravesical 'cough spike'

## Comment

Urethral pressure profilometry has enjoyed a disproportionate amount of attention. The results obtained are extremely susceptible to experimental artefacts and the patient's degree of relaxation and in addition this study can be distressingly uncomfortable for patients, especially males.

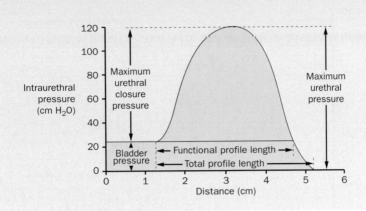

**Figure 3.23  Diagram of a female urethral pressure profile in storage phase with the nomenclature recommended by the International Continence Society.**
(Reproduced with permission from Neurourology and Urodynamics 1988; 7:403–426.)

The information gained from urethral pressure measurements in the storage phase is of limited value in the assessment of voiding disorders. Total profile length is not generally regarded as a useful parameter.

The VUPP is not yet fully developed as a technique and a number of technical and clinical problems need to be solved before it is widely used.

## AMBULATORY URODYNAMICS

Conventional urodynamics is nonphysiological and can be insensitive because it may not equate with clinical diagnoses. From the literature it appears that detrusor instability is actually detected using a conventional study in only about 50% of patients who have symptoms highly suggestive of detrusor instability. Despite this, conventional urodynamics is the present day 'gold standard' investigation of lower urinary tract dysfunction.

Ambulatory urodynamic monitoring overcomes some of these limitations with natural bladder filling and the patient is fully ambulant and able to carry out everyday activities, which may provoke symptoms.

The idea and technique parallel those for ambulatory monitoring of the cadiovascular and gastrointestinal systems, but have been slower to gain acceptance for urological investigation. After initial enthusiasm in the 1960s it was largely abandoned until the late 1980s. Since then, it has become more popular, but whether this is appropriate for widespread clinical use is debatable.

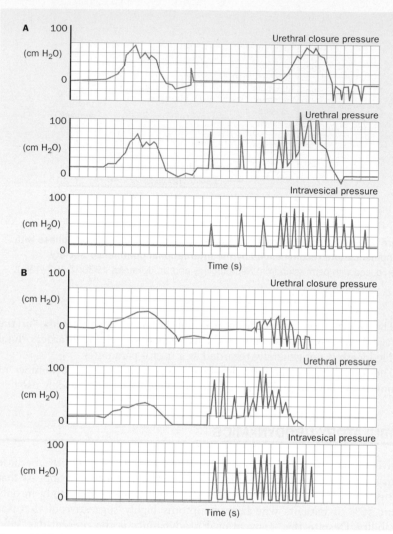

**Figure 3.24 Pressure 'transmission' ratio.** (A) Urethral pressure profiles in a normal female at rest (on the left) and while coughing (on the right). During coughing there is transmission of intra-abdominal pressure (represented by the bladder trace) to the urethra in all except the distal portion of the profile. (B) Urethral pressure profiles in a patient who has genuine stress incontinence at rest (on the left) and while coughing (on the right). At rest the bladder pressure trace is flattened compared with normal and during coughing there is a lack of the normal transmission of intra-abdominal pressure to the urethra, resulting in negative deflections in the urethral closure pressure trace. This abnormal response results from a prolapse of the urethra within a cystourethrocoele. (Reproduced from Abrams P, Feneley R, and Torrens M, Urodynamics. Berlin: Springer; 1983.)

The basic equipment needed for ambulatory monitoring comprises:
- vesical and rectal catheters (either fluid filled or microtransducers) to measure pressures;
- a portable storage device to record data; and
- a PC for processing and plotting the data.

Most storage devices are battery powered and allow information to be collected for several hours. Extra channels on the devices collect measurements of urine loss and, more recently, of simultaneous flow rate data (Figures 3.25 and 3.26).

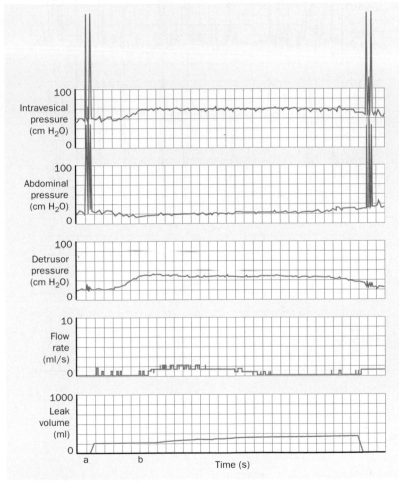

**Figure 3.25  Typical AUM trace demonstrating sequence of (a) cough test (b) voluntary void.**

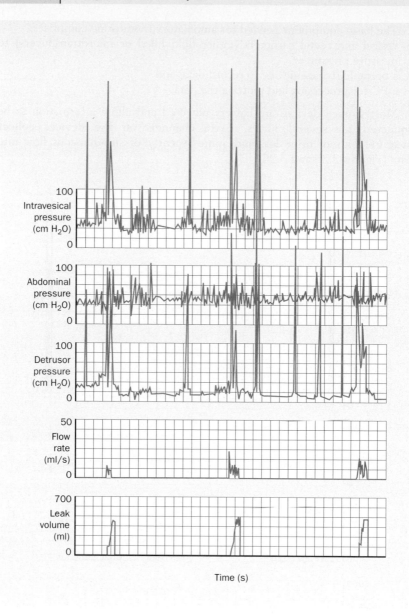

**Figure 3.26 Obstructed subject.** Full trace including 3 voids.

Differences in filling and voiding parameters have been identified by comparison with conventional cystometry using artificial 'filling' in both normal volunteers and symptomatic patients. For ambulatory urodynamics these comparisons show.

• lower pressure increases during filling, even in patients who have low compliance on conventional monitoring;
• increased amplitude of voiding pressures;
• similar or reduced voided volumes;
• increased ability to diagnose a functional abnormality associated with incontinence; and
• increased ability to detect uninhibited detrusor activity.

The explanation for these apparent differences between ambulatory and conventional urodynamics may relate to the circumstances associated with the ambulatory test. In particular, it is not physiological to have catheters *in situ* for 3 4 hours.

Some of the voiding parameters may be explained by less overfilling of the bladder due to the slower fill and therefore they may be more closely correlated with the actual functional bladder capacity (Figure 3.26).

Medium and fast fill may be too insensitive, being too fast to allow detection of 'normal' or 'pathological' detrusor activity.

An explanation of these differences is awaited following ongoing research involving asymptomatic volunteers and patients who have lower urinary tract dysfunction. Ambulatory urodynamics should not be used as a routine clinical investigation until the ranges of 'normality' for this technique have been adequately defined.

## ELECTROMYOGRAPHY

Electromyography (EMG) is the study of electrical potentials generated by the depolarization of muscle, and in this context refers to urethral sphincter striated muscle EMG. The functional unit in EMG is the motor unit. This is comprised of a single motor neurone and the muscle fibres and results from activation of a single anterior horn cell (Figure 3.27). Muscle action potentials can be detected either by needle or surface electrodes.

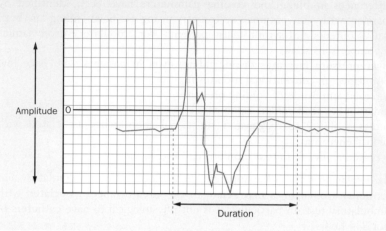

**Figure 3.27   Muscle action potential from a urethral sphincter electromyogram.**

## URODYNAMICS IN PRACTICE: ELECTROMYOGRAPHY

### Needle electrodes (concentric, bipolar, monopolar, single fibre)
- These are placed directly into the muscle mass and allow visualization of the individual motor unit action potentials (see Figure 3.27)

### Surface electrodes (skin, anal plug, catheter)
- Are applied to an epithelial surface as close to the muscle being studied as possible
- Detect the action potentials from groups of adjacent motor units underlying the recording surface
- Can be difficult to secure adequately and provide less reproducible results than needle electrodes

### Practical points
The EMG potentials can be displayed on an oscilloscope screen or played through audio amplifiers. A permanent record of EMG potentials can only be made using a chart recorder with a high-frequency response (in the range of 10 kHz).

A skilled investigator is needed to interpret needle EMG results.

### Comment
The EMG should be interpreted in the light of the patient's symptoms, physical findings, and urological and urodynamic investigations.

The main clinical indication for EMG studies is as an adjunct to videocystometrography to distinguish between striated and smooth muscle in neuropathic-type distal urethral obstruction.

Other EMG studies provide interesting scientific information, but this rarely alters the clinical management of patients.

## NERVE CONDUCTION STUDIES

Nerve conduction studies involve:
* stimulation of a peripheral nerve; and
* recording the time for a response to occur in muscle innervated by the nerve under study.

## REFLEX LATENCIES

Reflex latencies require:
* stimulation of sensory fields; and
* recordings from the muscle that contracts reflexly in response to the stimulation.

Such responses are a test of the reflex arcs, which are comprised of both afferent and efferent limbs and the synapses within the CNS.

The reflex latency expresses:
* the nerve conduction velocity in both limbs of the reflex arc; and
* the integrity of the CNS at the level of the synapse(s).

Increased reflex latency may result from slowed afferent or efferent nerve conduction or delayed CNS conduction.

## SENSORY TESTING

Limited subjective information may be obtained during cystometry by recording parameters such as the first desire to micturate, urgency, or pain. Sensory function in the lower urinary tract can also be assessed by semi-objective tests that rely upon the measurement of urethral or vesical sensory thresholds to a standard applied stimulus such as a known electrical current.

### Bladder and urethral sensory thresholds
These are defined as the least current that consistently produces a sensation perceived by the subject during stimulation at the site under investigation. The absolute values vary in relation to the site of the stimulus, the characteristics of the equipment, and the stimulation parameters.

## UPPER URINARY TRACT URODYNAMICS – THE WHITAKER TEST

Upper urinary tract obstruction often goes unrecognised. The clinical indications for functional studies are chronic loin pain or deteriorating renal function where an obstructing ureteric lesion has not been excluded or where the significance of an obstructing lesion is in doubt.

Diuresis excretory urography by itself has little use because anatomical demonstration of a dilated system neither confirms nor excludes obstruction. The techniques now used to investigate equivocally obstructed kidneys are:

- diuresis renography;
- radionuclide parenchymal transit times; and
- pressure–flow studies.

Nuclear medicine studies are particularly important for providing an assessment of differential renal function and are essential in serial follow-up.

The upper urinary tract is a highly distensible system that is normally protected from the intermittent high pressure generated by the bladder by the competent vesicoureteric junction. Under normal circumstances:

- urine accumulates in the renal pelvis at a resting pressure of less than 5 cm $H_2O$;
- the pelvic pressure rises to 10 cm $H_2O$ on distension; and
- urine enters the ureter to be transported as a bolus to the bladder by ureteric peristalsis at intra-bolus pressures of 20–60 cm $H_2O$.

Efficient peristalsis is dependent upon apposition of the ureteric walls. Ureteric dilatation (whether obstructive or not) and disorders of wall mobility prevent the ureteric walls opposing, compromising the efficiency of urine transport and tubular flow.

The normal response of the upper urinary tract to obstruction at or above the vesicoureteric junction is:

- an increase in the rate of ureteric and pelvic peristalsis; and
- eventual ureteric dilatation.

Ureteric dilatation causes discoordinated peristalsis and inefficient urine transport. As flow is reduced down the ureter, pressure rises are transmitted:

- first to the collecting ducts; and
- then along the tubules to the glomeruli.

If there is no parallel increase in the glomerular hydrostatic pressure, filtration will eventually stop.

Pressure–flow studies involve perfusion of the kidney with contrast at a known rate while simultaneously measuring the pressure within the renal pelvis and bladder:

- significant rises in pressure are indicative of obstruction; whereas
- free drainage at low pressure excludes obstruction.

## URODYNAMICS IN PRACTICE: THE WHITAKER TEST

- Performed under local anaesthesia following premedication with diazepam unless the patient has an indwelling nephrostomy catheter
- Bladder pressure is measured via a urethral catheter connected to a transducer
- Renal pelvic pressure can be measured through a nephrostomy tube or through a needle placed in the collecting system at antegrade pyelography – the puncture technique must be good because any leak from the collecting system degrades the information provided by pressure studies
- Dilute contrast is infused through one arm of a 'Y' connector at an initial rate of 10 ml/min while the other arm of the 'Y' is connected to a pressure transducer recording renal pelvic pressure in response to perfusion (Figure 3.28) – perfusion at 10 ml/min is considerably in excess of physiological rates
- Bladder pressure is continuously recorded and the subtracted pressure (pelvic pressure – bladder pressure) is automatically calculated – appropriate manometric equipment is available in any department performing lower urinary tract urodynamics
- Simultaneous fluoroscopy defines the anatomy of the upper tract and spot films can be taken

### Practical points

Using this technique a pressure difference between the upper and lower urinary tract of:

- less than 15 cm $H_2O$ excludes obstruction;
- more than 22 cm $H_2O$, confirms obstruction; and
- 15–22 cm $H_2O$ lies in the equivocal range.

Vesicoureteral reflux has occurred if both the bladder and pelvic pressure increase equally together.

Higher rates of perfusion have been advocated, but their clinical usefulness is debatable.

Loin pain can occur in patients who have a urinary diversion (e.g. ileal loop) because of the high pressures generated by bowel peristalsis refluxing up the reinplanted ureters; the extent of this can be easily assessed by upper urinary tract urodynamics.

### Comment

The main value of upper urinary tract urodynamics is in providing an accurate objective assessment about whether there is obstruction to renal drainage.

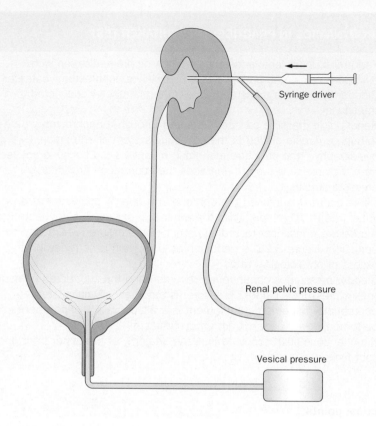

**Figure 3.28    Diagram of the Whitaker test.**

Upper urinary tract urodynamics is an invasive procedure because a percutaneous nephrostomy tract is required and so it should be reserved for cases where other investigations such as excretory urography and isotope renography have produced equivocal results.

## MICTURITION PROBLEMS IN UROLOGICAL PRACTICE

The major problems of micturition encountered in urological practice can be considered in three main groups:
- difficulty voiding;
- urinary incontinence; and
- voiding frequency.

A variety of aetiological factors can result in any one of these three symptoms and these are summarized in Figure 3.29.

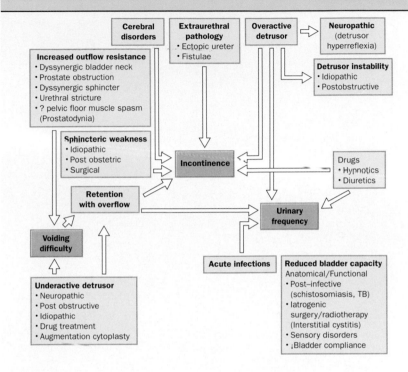

**Figure 3.29   Common urological symptoms and their aetiology.**

# FURTHER READING

It is clear that urodynamic evaluation is essential for the accurate investigation of patients who have lower urinary tract symptoms. Because only a brief summary of this subject can be provided here, comprehensive reviews should be consulted for more detailed information:

Abrams P. Urodynamics, 2nd ed. London: Springer-Verlag; 1997.

Abrams P, Griffiths D, Buzelin JM, et al. The urodynamic assessment of lower urinary tract symptoms. In: Denis L, Griffiths K, Khoury S, et al., eds. 4th International Consultation on BPH, Proceedings. Plymouth: Health Publication; 1998:325.

Mundy AR, Stephenson TP, Wein AJ, eds. Urodynamics – principles, practice and application, 2nd ed. Edinburgh: Churchill Livingstone; 1994.

## INTRODUCTION

Voiding difficulty is the commonest reason for men to present to urologists because of the common prevalence of prostatic outflow obstruction in males. Voiding difficulty is an uncommon reason for referral of women to a urologist. Most female patients with voiding difficulty have a neuropathic disorder affecting the bladder.

Causes of voiding difficulty in men are:

- increased outflow resistance (most cases) resulting from obstruction at the level of the bladder neck or prostate or a urethral stricture; and
- detrusor muscle failure (occasional cases), which may be either primary or secondary to the outflow obstruction.

## URETHRAL STRICTURE

Urethral stricture usually occurs in males, who present with a history of:
- diminished stream (once the urethral calibre is reduced below 11 F); and
- a prolonged slow flow rate.

Once suspected a urethral stricture is best demonstrated by urethrography.

Therapy consists of urethral dilatation, urethrotomy or urethroplasty.

## PROSTATIC OBSTRUCTION

Both benign and malignant enlargement of the prostate are increasingly common with advancing age in elderly men. Terminology relating to enlargement of the prostate includes:

- benign prostatic hyperplasia (BPH), which is a histological diagnosis and present in up to 50% of men over 60 years of age and nearly 88% by 80 years of age – the extent to which symptoms secondary to BPH manifest themselves is variable;
- benign prostatic enlargement (BPE) – the macroscopically demonstrable growth of the gland; and
- bladder outflow obstruction (BOO) – the urodynamically proven obstruction to the passage of urine.

It has been estimated that 25% of men in their sixth decade have urinary symptoms and objective signs of BOO.

Only 60–70% of patients who have typical symptoms of BOO have proven obstruction on urodynamic studies, and the term lower urinary tract symptoms (LUTS) is therefore preferable to 'prostatism', which implies a disease specificity for symptoms.

Prostatic adenocarcinoma is the most common tumour of the male genitourinary tract.

Benign and malignant prostatic disease often coexist, but the relationship appears to be coincidental. Although both conditions are under the trophic influence of the male hormone testosterone:

- carcinoma usually originates in the peripheral zone of the gland; and
- benign adenomas in the periurethral central zone.

Symptoms of bladder overactivity characterized by detrusor instability occur in up to 70% of men who present with prostatic outflow obstruction and are more common with increasing age. It resolves following surgical relief of the obstruction in up to two-thirds of patients, which suggests a causal link between detrusor instability and outlet obstruction in some patients.

Acute retention is common and usually makes a marked contribution to the clinical workload of a urologist in a district general hospital. Usually it occurs in a patient who has a pre-existing history of prostatic outflow obstruction. Acute retention may be precipitated by increased sympathetic stimulation acting upon the bladder and outflow tract, particularly the prostatic urethra. Common precipitating factors implicated are:

- stress, physical or mental;
- alcohol consumption;
- a cold environmental temperature; and
- constipation.

**History and examination**

Lower urinary tract symptoms can be subdivided into two main groups:

- storage symptoms – the overactive bladder – frequency, nocturia, urgency, with or without urge incontinence; and
- voiding symptoms – hesitancy, poor stream, feeling of incomplete bladder emptying.

Because only 60–70% of patients who have typical symptoms of BOO have proven obstruction, the term LUTS is preferred to describe these symptoms rather than prostatism. In addition, although it is tempting to equate detrusor instability as being synonymous with irritant symptoms, no such causal relationship has yet been established. An overview for the assessment of patients with LUTS is given in Figure 4.1.

## Assessment of lower urinary tract symptoms

| Aspect | Relevant information or investigations | Notes |
|---|---|---|
| Symptoms and quality of life | Urinary symptoms | Document previous treatment. Assess degree of bother (International Prostate Symptom Score, Figure 4.2); enquire about haematuria, neurological disease, medication, polyuria, urinary tract infection, frequency and urgency |
| Physical examination | General examination, abdominal examination, pelvic examination, digital rectal examination and focused neurological examination | Digital rectal examination is essential Pelvic examination will illustrate possible uterine/ovarian abnormalities |
| Uroflowmetry | Determine maximum flow rate, flow pattern, and volumes voided; flow rates vary, so obtain at least two voids of preferably >150ml | Patients who have BOO tend to produce a typical flow pattern with a delayed and reduced maximum flow rate; generally, BOO is likely if maximum flow rate <10ml/s, but unlikely if flow rate >15ml/s; a slow flow may be due to detrusor underactivity, especially when associated with an increased postmicturition residual volume |
| Post-micturition residual volumes | Obtained using transabdominal ultrasonography /catheterization | Incomplete emptying reduces functional bladder capacity and may account for symptoms or the propensity to develop complications; an increase in residual urine volume is a sign of bladder decompensation rather than obstruction |
| Other urological tests | Renal function<br><br>Urinalysis | Bladder outflow obstruction may contribute to renal failure Exclude urinary tract infection, haematuria indicating possible bladder tumour, proteinuria, glycosuria |
| Tests for prostate cancer | Total PSA | Use of this assay is controversial – essentially, it is recommended either for patients who would be suitable for radical prostate surgery and radiotherapy if a localized prostate cancer is diagnosed or to augment equivocal digital rectal findings |

**Figure 4.1  Assessment of lower urinary tract symptoms.** (BOO, bladder outflow obstruction; PSA, prostate-specific antigen.)

## Assessment of lower urinary tract symptoms

| Aspect | Relevant information or investigations | Notes |
|---|---|---|
| Tests for prostate cancer (*contd*) | Transrectal ultrasonography | Used to aid in diagnosis of prostate cancer and to guide prostate biopsy; it is also helpful in determining prostate size and morphology, which may influence treatment options |
| | Prostate biopsy | Required to make the histological diagnosis of prostate cancer |
| Invasive urological tests | Cystometry and VCMG Allow observation of sensory and motor function of the bladder during filling, but cystometry is invasive | The relationship between voiding detrusor pressure and flow rate allows classification of various degrees of obstruction; the presence of documented obstruction usually leads to a satisfactory outcome in 90% of patients; operative management of patients who do not have obstruction leads to less than optimal results; cystometry is restricted to selected patients – younger patients who have predominant filling symptoms or have underlying neuropathology, those who have had previous prostate surgery, and to determine detrusor function |
| | Cystoscopy | Reserved for patients who have suspected underlying intravesical pathology, including patients who have predominant filling symptoms, haematuria, and repeated urinary tract infections |

**Figure 4.1 Assessment of lower urinary tract symptoms** (*contd*).
(VCMG, videocystometrogram.)

**International Prostate Symptom Score (I-PSS)**    *(Please circle the appropriate score)*

|  | Not at all | Less than 1 time in 5 | Less than half the time | About half the time | More than half the time | Almost always |
|---|---|---|---|---|---|---|
| 1. Since the last visit, how often have you had a sensation of not emptying your bladder completely after you finished urinating? | 0 | 1 | 2 | 3 | 4 | 5 |
| 2. Since the last visit, how often have you had to urinate again less than two hours after you finished urinating? | 0 | 1 | 2 | 3 | 4 | 5 |
| 3. Since the last visit, how often have you found you stopped and started again several times when you urinated? | 0 | 1 | 2 | 3 | 4 | 5 |
| 4. Since the last visit, how often have you found it difficult to postpone urination? | 0 | 1 | 2 | 3 | 4 | 5 |
| 5. Since the last visit, how often have you had a weak urinary stream? | 0 | 1 | 2 | 3 | 4 | 5 |
| 6. Since the last visit, how often have you had to push or strain to begin urination? | 0 | 1 | 2 | 3 | 4 | 5 |
|  | None | 1 time | 2 times | 3 times | 4 times | 5 or more times |
| 7. Since the last visit, how many times did you most typically get up to urinate from the time you went to bed at night until the time you got up in the morning? | 0 | 1 | 2 | 3 | 4 | 5 |

**Total I-PS Score, S=**

**Quality of life due to urinary symptoms**    *(Please circle the appropriate score)*

|  | Delighted | Pleased | Mostly satisfied | Mixed (about equally satisfied and dissatisfied) | Mostly dissatisfied | Unhappy | Terrible |
|---|---|---|---|---|---|---|---|
| 1. If you were to spend the rest of your life with your urinary condition just the way it is now, how would you feel about that? | 0 | 1 | 2 | 3 | 4 | 5 | 6 |

**Quality of life assessment score =**

**Figure 4.2   International Prostate Symptom Score.**

The symptom of postmicturition dribble is not due to obstruction, but results from bulbar pooling and is therefore common:
- in elderly men;
- in association with a urethral stricture or following urethroplasty; and
- if there is bladder neck obstruction.

Clinical examination may reveal a palpable bladder and thereby confirm a diagnosis of urinary retention. Digital rectal examination is essential because this may reveal a malignant neoplasm and transrectal ultrasound with biopsy can be useful in confirming this.

## URODYNAMICS IN PRACTICE: PROSTATIC OBSTRUCTION

- In most cases a flow rate and urinary residual volume estimation are sufficient to confirm a diagnosis of prostatic obstruction
- Normal voiding can be maintained during the early stages of prostatic obstruction by a compensatory increase in voiding detrusor pressure
- Flow rate will not be able to differentiate between high pressure with low flow and low pressure with low flow – this distinction is important because many patients who have an unsatisfactory result following previous prostatic surgery have low pressure with low flow
- More detailed urodynamic investigation is therefore essential if the flow rate is equivocal or previous surgery has not led to any improvement or left residual symptoms such as incontinence (to differentiate between detrusor instability and sphincteric weakness)
- Typical cystometrogram (CMG) and videocystometrogram (VCMG) appearances are demonstrated in Figure 4.3.

### Management
In the past decade several alternatives to prostatectomy have been developed for the treatment of BPH. The mechanism of action of these treatments is to shrink the prostate or relax the smooth muscle within the gland. These can be broadly categorized into medical and surgical techniques.

The objectives of treatment are to:
- relieve symptoms and improve quality of life;
- relieve bladder obstruction;
- prevent and treat complications resulting from BOO.

The various treatment modalities – pharmacotherapy, minimally invasive procedures, and surgical prostatectomy – are not comparable in terms of efficacy or invasiveness so this is where there is an element of choice, bearing in mind the potential advantages and disadvantages of each therapy. Most patients given the choice opt for either watchful waiting or pharmacotherapy.

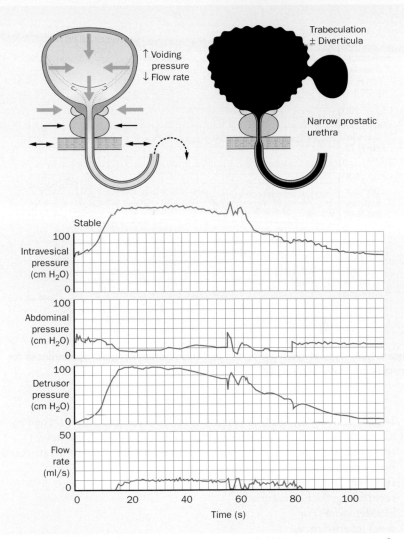

**Figure 4.3A   Typical cystometrogram and videocystometrogram appearances for stable prostatic obstruction.**

**81**

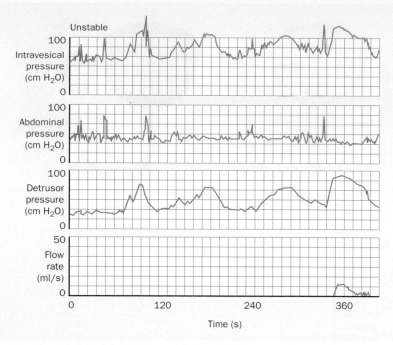

**Figure 4.3B  Typical cystometrogram and videocystometrogram appearances for unstable prostatic obstruction.**

It is generally accepted that patients who have complications secondary to BOO should be treated operatively. This includes patients who have:
- refractory urinary retention who have failed a trial without a catheter at least once;
- recurrent urinary tract infections;
- recurrent gross haematuria;
- bladder stones; or
- renal insufficiency.

An algorithm for the management of LUTS due to bladder outflow obstruction is given in Figure 4.4.

### Watchful waiting
Not all patients who have untreated BPH deteriorate. A meta-analysis of existing studies has shown that the symptoms of 16% of those who have BPH do not change and nearly 40% improve with a follow-up ranging from 2.6–5 years. In this context a policy of watchful waiting has been advocated for patients who have mild or moderate symptoms.

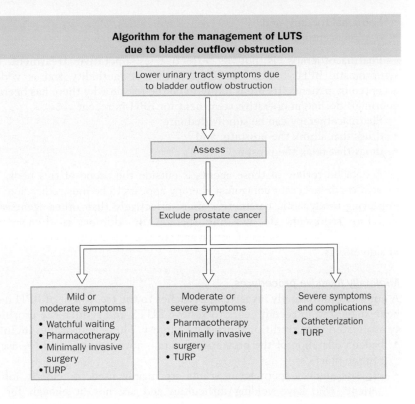

**Figure 4.4  Algorithm for the management of LUTS due to bladder outflow obstruction.** (TURP, transurethral resection of prostate.)

Generally the disease progression is slow. It is prudent for patients to be monitored periodically to check that there has been no marked deterioration.

### Pharmacotherapy

In recent years it has become clear that pharmacotherapy can be beneficial. The primary indications for pharmacotherapy are:
- symptomatic patients who desire therapy and who do not have an indication for surgery;
- patients who decline operative management;
- medical conditions that contraindicate operative management; and
- as an interim treatment while awaiting operation.

Three classes of drugs have been used for the medical management of BPH:
- phytotherapy;

- hormonal therapy; and
- α-adrenoceptor antagonists.

Pharmacotherapy is not as effective as operative treatment for symptomatic BPH, but is associated with less morbidity and is widely accepted by patients. Its use is likely to be the reason why there has been an enormous decline in operative treatment for BPH in recent years.

Pharmacotherapy can be subdivided into:
- drugs that shrink the prostate; and
- drugs that relax the prostate.

A detailed review of these agents is outside the scope of this book. At present α-adrenoceptor antagonist therapy appears to be most efficacious by improving urodynamic parameters more effectively than other agents and therefore represents the first-line therapy. In addition, α-adrenoceptor antagonists have a fast onset of action and are associated with a tolerable level of side effects.

### Minimally invasive procedures

A number of minimally invasive approaches to the treatment of BPH have been suggested in recent years to relieve LUTS and reduce the morbidity associated with traditional prostate surgery. These approaches include:
- balloon dilatation of the prostatic urethra – not recommended for use in routine practice;
- prostate stents – permanent stents are mainly used for elderly infirm patients who have voiding difficulties and are not fit enough for an operation and those who do not wish to have long-term catheterization;
- high intensity focused ultrasound (HIFU) – under evaluation;
- transurethral microwave thermotherapy (TUMT) – the improvements in urodynamic parameters have tended to be less than those observed with transurethral resection of the prostate (TURP);
- transurethral needle ablation of the prostate (TUNA) – symptomatic improvement and increased flow rates have been reported;
- laser prostatectomy – visual laser ablation of the prostate (VLAP), contact laser ablation, interstitial laser therapy, laser excision of the prostate – advantages include minimal bleeding, a lower incidence of retrograde ejaculation and erectile dysfunction than following TURP, and it is safe to use for patients who are on anticoagulants;
- transurethral incision of the prostate (TUIP) – generally used for smaller prostates and involves incising the bladder neck to the level of the verumontanum down through the prostate into the perivesical fat; the associated morbidity is much less than that of TURP; and
- transurethral electrovaporization of the prostate – efficacy is reported to be similar to that obtained by TURP, and there may be a reduced associated morbidity in smaller glands.

A recent trend has been to combine electrovapourization with TURP using specially modified resection loops and this technique shows promise for the future.

With most of these minimally invasive treatments no tissue can be obtained for histology. There is a reported incidence of unsuspected prostate cancer being demonstrated histologically in up to 14% of cases following TURP, (though this percentage is likely to be less now because of the use of preoperative assessment with prostate-specific antigen and transrectal ultrasound of the prostate).

The efficacy, durability of treatment, and reoperation rates associated with these treatments must be considered. Recent reports indicate that there is a higher reoperation rate compared with that following TURP. Certainly at present these 'new' minimally invasive alternatives comprise significantly less than 10% of the surgical procedures for symptomatic patients with LUTS secondary to BOO.

### Surgical options – prostatectomy
#### Transurethral resection of the prostate

This procedure has stood the test of time and remains the most effective treatment for bladder outflow obstruction secondary to BPH. It is performed under regional or general anaesthetic. The prostate is resected electrosurgically, creating a cavity. The prostate chips are evacuated and the bladder is irrigated via a catheter. The catheter is removed when the bleeding settles.

Complications associated with TURP include:

- haemorrhage with or without clot retention – about 10% of all cases that undergo operation require a blood transfusion;
- fluid absorption resulting in the transurethral resection syndrome – reported in 1% of cases;
- infection – 1–2% of cases;
- incontinence – 1–2% of cases;
- urethral stricture and bladder neck stenosis – late complications that occur in 3–16% of cases;
- retrograde ejaculation – occurs in most cases; and
- deterioration in erectile function in up to 25% of cases.

Outcome studies indicate that patients who have severe symptoms preoperatively show the greatest improvements in symptoms and quality of life, with over 90% of such men reporting an improvement compared with less than 80% of men who had moderate symptoms. The overall operative mortality has been quoted as 0.5–1% and the mortality rate increases with increasing patient age, and is higher in these patients presenting with urinary retention.

*Retropubic prostatectomy*

Open prostatectomy is restricted to those few patients who have very large prostates. In this context an open prostatectomy is quicker and safer.

*Catheterization*

Patients who have detrusor underactivity (see below) may develop chronic retention and their symptoms are less likely to resolve following a prostate operation. In these cases the bladder needs to be emptied either by:

- intermittent self-catheterization; or
- an indwelling catheter (preferably suprapubic).

Intermittent self-catheterization is the preferred option because catheter-related complications are then minimized if hygiene and compliance are adequate. Consideration can be given to proceeding to prostatectomy if there is evidence of recovery of detrusor function.

---

### SUMMARY: PROSTATIC OBSTRUCTION

- Evaluation of a patient who has symptomatic BPH includes obtaining an appropriate history, physical examination, urinalysis, laboratory tests, and uroflowmetry
- Treatment is directed at improving quality of life, relieving BOO, and resolving BOO complications
- Watchful waiting and pharmacotherapy tend to be the choice of therapy for mild to moderate symptoms
- Minimally invasive procedures cause less morbidity (at least half that of TURP in the short term), but are less effective and durable, so TURP remains the 'gold standard' technique
- Many patients prefer a nonoperative therapy, so in recent years there has been an enormous decline in the number of prostate operations carried out

---

## OBSTRUCTION DUE TO URETHRAL OVERACTIVITY

During normal voiding the urethra relaxes synchronously with contraction of the detrusor muscle. Should the urethra and in particular its associated sphincter mechanisms fail to relax, dysfunctional voiding occurs. The three main types of such dysfunctional voiding are:

- failure of the bladder neck mechanism to relax – detrusor–bladder neck dyssynergia, otherwise known as bladder neck obstruction;
- detrusor–sphincter dyssynergia which complicates a number of neurological disorders affecting the lower urinary tract – commonly Parkinson's disease and multiple sclerosis; and

- detrusor–urethral dyssynergia – a little recognised condition primarily affecting young women in whom the urethral sphincter mechanism fails to relax.

## History and examination

The brief descriptions given above should be borne in mind when taking a history from any patient who has outflow obstruction. Associated neurological symptoms and signs should suggest the possibility of detrusor–sphincter dyssynergia.

### *Detrusor–bladder neck dyssynergia*

The patient who has detrusor–bladder neck dyssynergia usually presents with:
- voiding difficulty in the third decade of life; or
- a complication of outflow obstruction such as urinary tract infection.

Further questioning will often reveal a lifelong history of diminished urinary stream.

### *Detrusor–urethral dyssynergia*

This occurs in young women who present with a history of lifelong voiding difficulty and often there is associated secondary detrusor failure. Many of these women have an associated hormonal problem (Stein–Leventhal syndrome – hirsutism, polycystic ovaries, and amenorrhoea) and characteristic motor unit appearances on electromyography – the so-called Fowler syndrome.

---

**URODYNAMICS IN PRACTICE: OBSTRUCTION DUE TO URETHRAL OVERACTIVITY**

**Detrusor–sphincter dyssynergia**
- Best demonstrated on videocystometry (Figure 4.5) with the synchronous use of electromyography

**Detrusor–bladder neck dyssynergia**
- Videocystometry will demonstrate findings suggestive of bladder outflow obstruction and in particular will show the trapping of contrast at the bladder neck on carrying out a stop test (i.e. ask the patient to stop voiding voluntarily; Figures 3.11 and 4.6)
- We have recently found that a characteristic lucent area is invariably seen on transrectal ultrasound scans in the dorsal area of the bladder neck in these patients

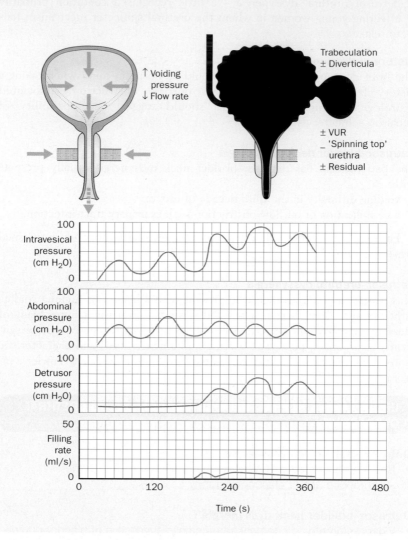

**Figure 4.5 Typical cystometrogram and videocystometrogram appearances for detrusor–sphincter dyssynergia.** VUR, vesicoureteral reflux. Note the intermittent straining pattern and high pressure low flow voiding parameters.

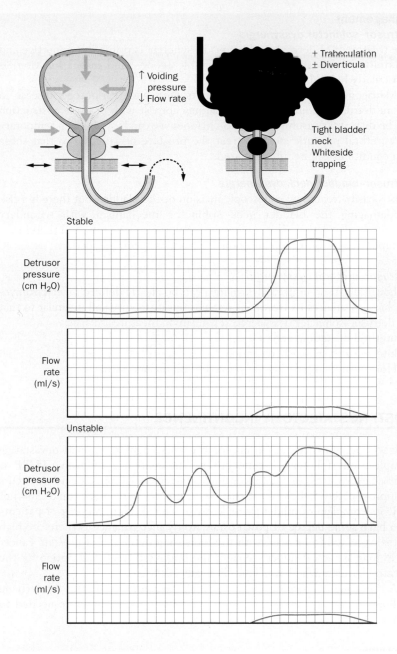

Figure 4.6   Typical cystometrogram and videocystometrogram appearances for detrusor–bladder neck dyssynergia.

## Management
### Detrusor–sphincter dyssynergia
The treatment of detrusor–sphincter dyssynergia is primarily supportive and intermittent self-catheterization if feasible (good hand motor function) is particularly helpful.

Management of elderly male patients who have Parkinson's disease in whom detrusor–sphincter dyssynergia may coexist with prostate obstruction can be difficult. A useful therapeutic manoeuvre can be to insert a temporary intraurethral prostatic stent to treat the prostate obstruction so that these two conditions can be differentiated.

### Detrusor–bladder neck dyssynergia
This is easily treated by endoscopic incision of the bladder, but there is a risk of damaging the bladder neck sphincter mechanism with secondary retrograde ejaculation. This can impair fertility in young men and therefore a therapeutic trial of $\alpha_1$-adrenoceptor blockade is recommended.

### Detrusor–urethral dyssynergia
Although detrusor–urethral dyssynergia can be clearly defined on electromyographic appearances its treatment remains unsatisfactory and is similar to that for detrusor–sphincter dyssynergia relying upon measures such as:
* urethral dilatation; and
* intermittent self-catheterization.
  Hormonal manipulation has proved to be unsuccessful.

## POSTPROSTATECTOMY INCONTINENCE

Urinary incontinence can be one of the most debilitating and devastating complications following prostatectomy. Its incidence following TURP is 2–5%. Severe stress or total incontinence after radical prostatectomy occurs in approximately 5–12% of patients, and a greater percentage (up to 50%) of patients complain of milder stress leakage. The absolute number of patients who have some degree of postprostatectomy incontinence is therefore high and is expected to increase with the increasing detection of prostate cancer for as long as radical surgery remains the preferred treatment option for the selected patients who have clinically localized disease.

A thorough knowledge of normal anatomy and the underlying pathophysiology of postprostatectomy incontinence is therefore needed to understand its investigation and management.

### Anatomy
In the male, continence relies upon the presence of two functionally independent sphincter mechanisms:

- the proximal (bladder neck) urethral sphincter; and
- distal (external) urethral sphincter.

The proximal sphincter is composed of smooth muscle and is ablated during a TURP or radical prostatectomy. The distal sphincter is confined to the 3–5 mm thickness of the wall of the membranous urethra from the level of the verumontanum down to the distal aspect of the membranous urethra. It is composed mainly of slow-twitch striated muscle fibres, which are capable of the sustained contraction necessary for continence. The distal sphincter maintains continence following a prostatectomy.

## Pathophysiology

Postprostatectomy incontinence can result from a variety of underlying pathological processes.

Distal sphincteric incompetence can precede or result from prostatectomy.

- predisposing causes of distal sphincteric damage before prostatectomy include pelvic trauma, denervation after radical pelvic surgery or intervertebral disc disease, and radical radiotherapy.
- sphincteric incompetence resulting from surgery is usually a result of direct injury or secondary to denervation or periurethral fibrosis.

The intrinsic smooth muscle distal sphincter mechanism is separate from the extrinsic skeletal muscle of the periurethral pelvic floor, explaining why most patients who have postprostatectomy incontinence are capable of stopping and starting their urinary stream.

Not all postprostatectomy incontinence is secondary to sphincteric incompetence. Obstruction resulting in overflow incontinence must be ruled out and may be secondary to a bladder neck contracture or urethral stricture.

Reduced bladder compliance and detrusor instability may be present in up to 50% of patients who are incontinent following prostatectomy and may be the underlying cause or a major contributing factor.

In many cases the bladder overactivity is present from the onset, but becomes problematical following prostatectomy as a consequence of the marked reduction in the integrity of the urethral sphincter mechanism.

## Investigation

Patients who present with incontinence following prostatectomy require an in-depth history and physical examination. Most patients give a history of stress incontinence and slow dribbling leakage when standing upright. Many patients are continent when supine and only experience urge incontinence when changing posture to the standing position.

Patients who have sphincteric incompetence leak when asked to carry out a Valsalva manoeuvre.

Overflow incontinence can be diagnosed by suprapubic palpation and measuring a postvoid residual urine volume. An abnormal neurological examination may suggest an underlying abnormality leading to sphincteric denervation.

Urinalysis is necessary to test for urinary tract infection.

## URODYNAMICS IN PRACTICE: POSTPROSTATECTOMY INCONTINENCE

- The cornerstone for evaluating incontinence following prostatectomy
- Will establish a diagnosis of sphincteric incompetence
- Will identify and characterize bladder dysfunction, which may be observed either in isolation or in combination with impaired sphincter function
- Following prostatectomy commonly demonstrate poor bladder compliance, bladder instability, and bladder hypersensitivity
- Demonstration of stress incontinence during urodynamics is necessary to diagnose sphincteric incompetence – a low abdominal leak point pressure of less than 60 cm $H_2O$ correlates with sphincteric incompetence, but is not diagnostic
- Measurement of the urethral pressure profile is of limited value and is generally not recommended
- Simultaneous measurement of voiding pressure and flow combined with radiological screening help to identify the presence and site of obstruction as well as detrusor hypocontractility
- Measurement of residual urine volume following free uroflow is necessary to rule out overflow incontinence

## Management

Treatment of bladder dysfunction with pharmacotherapy and behavioural therapy is recommended before considering operative intervention. In addition, bladder overactivity that cannot be controlled medically is a poor prognositic indicator before insertion of an artificial urinary sphincter.

The therapeutic armamentarium for postprostatectomy incontinence includes:

- pharmacotherapy;
- periurethral injection therapy; and
- implantation of an artificial urinary sphincter.

Anticholinergic agents combined with a bladder drill are recommended for patients who have bladder overactivity and urge incontinence. Kegel's pelvic floor exercises play a limited role, but are encouraged, especially in the first few months postoperatively.

Periurethral injections include Macroplastique™, polytetrafluoroethylene and collagen. Continence is achieved by coaptation of the urethra proximal to the external sphincter and preferentially above the area of the anastomosis between the bladder and urethra (after radical prostatectomy), but the success rate is less than 30% and is significantly inferior to that obtained using artificial urinary sphincters.

The artificial urinary sphincter is the treatment of choice for stress incontinence secondary to sphincteric incompetence following prostatectomy. Approximately 90% of patients achieve social continence and nearly 50% achieve dryness. In experienced hands, the artificial urinary sphincter therefore gives patients the highest chance of cure and should be offered to appropriate patients.

## DETRUSOR FAILURE (UNDERACTIVE DETRUSOR FUNCTION)

Hypocontractile detrusor function should be considered for any patient who presents with voiding difficulty. It must always be suspected in any patient who presents with incontinence, particularly the elderly male for whom the diagnosis may be chronic retention with overflow incontinence. Objective demonstration of detrusor failure depends upon the use of formal cystometry.

### Chronic retention
This refers to a chronically distended bladder, whether resulting from:
- a known pathology such as prostate obstruction;
- urethral stricture; or
- a lower motor neurone lesion affecting the bladder.

Chronic retention often has an idiopathic aetiology and many patients who present with chronic retention in the presence of presumed prostatic obstruction in fact have a small prostate gland and may have an unidentified underlying predisposition to develop chronic retention.

A small but distinct group of middle-aged elderly female patients present with acute retention of urine, usually after surgery, and commonly vigorously deny any previous history of voiding difficulty. It is, however, possible to elicit a previous history of infrequent voiding ('camel bladder') for some of these patients. Urodynamic investigation demonstrates an underactive detrusor with chronic retention.

### URODYNAMICS IN PRACTICE: DETRUSOR FAILURE

- The urodynamic appearances of detrusor hypocontractivity are demonstrated in Figure 4.7

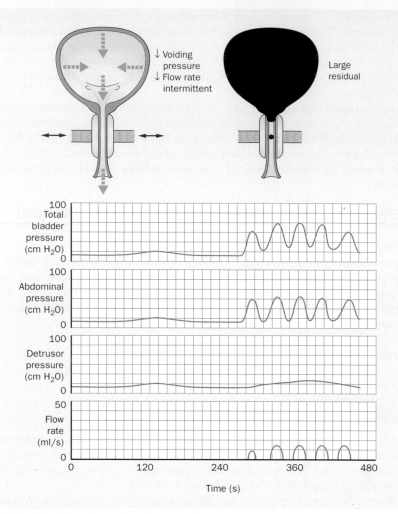

**Figure 4.7** Typical cystometrogram and videocystometrogram appearances for an underactive detrusor.

## Management

Correction of the underactive detrusor is aimed at correction of any underlying aetiology. In men, in the absence of a neurological deficit, it is presumed that there is a relative obstruction at the prostate level.

Therapeutic measures are as follows:

• ensuring that the bladder is emptied regularly to prevent back pressure and subsequent damage to the upper tracts by, in the majority of cases, using intermittent self-catheterization.

**94**

Placement of a suprapubic catheter, particularly in patients who have a neurological deficit that is potentially reversible, is important because:
- it decompresses the detrusor, preventing any further damage by over-distension of the detrusor muscle fibres; and
- allows careful assessment of postvoiding intravesical residual volumes.

Long-term therapeutic measures include:
- intermittent self-catheterization; and
- pharmacotherapy aimed at relaxing the outflow tract (e.g. $\alpha_1$-adrenoceptor antagonists).

Bladder training can be useful, particularly for the infrequent voiders who are instructed to void by the clock (e.g. 2-hourly).

Follow-up of patients is facilitated by careful monitoring of intravesical residual volumes using ultrasound (the ultrasound cystodynamogram, see p. 31).

# Chapter 5 | Incontinence

## INTRODUCTION

Urinary incontinence is defined as the involuntary leakage of urine that represents a social or hygienic problem and is objectively demonstrable. It is a symptom or sign, but not a diagnosis. The urinary leakage may be through:
- the urethra; or
- an extraurethral route or channel.

Urinary leakage through an extraurethral route may be congenital, as found with ectopic ureter, or iatrogenic as in vesicovaginal fistula. Incontinence affects millions of people worldwide, 85% of whom are women. Estimates indicate that as many as 1 in 4 women experience incontinence during their lifetime. More than one-third of healthy elderly women and approximately 50% of institutionalized females suffer from incontinence.

## TYPES OF INCONTINENCE

### Stress incontinence
Stress incontinence is the involuntary loss of urine associated with activities that increase intra-abdominal pressure such as coughing, sneezing, lifting, and physical exertion. In females, stress incontinence is usually associated with loss of pelvic floor support, resulting in descent or hypermobility of the bladder neck and proximal urethra but may also be due to intrinsic sphincter deficiency; indeed some degree of intrinsic sphincter deficiency is present in all female patients with stress incontinence. In men, stress incontinence is most commonly seen in patients following a radical prostatectomy. When the bladder descends, increases in intra-abdominal pressure are not transmitted equally to the bladder body and proximal urethra, but only to the bladder. This elevates intravesical pressure above the maximum pressure exerted by the urethral sphincter mechanism, resulting in stress incontinence.

### Urge incontinence
Urge incontinence is the involuntary loss of urine associated with a strong desire or urge to urinate. Patients usually complain of urinary frequency and nocturia as well.
Urge incontinence is:

- often associated with an involuntary increase in intravesical pressure during bladder filling – referred to as an unstable bladder contraction and sometimes inappropriately referred to as a 'bladder spasm';
- also seen in those who have poor bladder compliance or a hypersensitive bladder resulting in a small functional bladder capacity.
- approximately 30% of patients with frequency and urgency have a normal cystometrogram.

## Overflow incontinence

This is the involuntary loss of urine associated with overdistension of the bladder resulting from inefficient bladder emptying. It may occur as a result of:
- poor detrusor contractility;
- bladder outlet obstruction; or
- a combination of the two.

Overflow incontinence is uncommon in women but it is often seen in elderly men with chronic retention. Patients with inefficient bladder emptying and overdistension may present with unconscious dribbling, urinary frequency and urgency, or stress urinary incontinence. For this reason determination of the post-void residual urine volume is important in all patients with urinary incontinence.

## Unconscious incontinence

Unconscious involuntary incontinence is urine loss neither related to abdominal straining nor associated with urgency. The patient's first sensation is wetness. Its identification is important because it usually represents marked bladder dysfunction.

Most patients who have unconscious incontinence have either:
- marked intrinsic sphincter deficiency; or
- bladder instability not perceived as urgency because of poor bladder sensation (commonly seen in elderly patients and in those who have neuropathic bladders)
- overflow incontinence (uncommon in women, more common in men).

## Coexistence of different types of incontinence

Any of the types of incontinence described above can exist in combination. Many women who have stress incontinence due to urethrovesical hypermobility have an element of intrinsic sphincter deficiency or detrusor instability.

Identification of the various contributory factors is important because it influences treatment selection and helps in anticipating postoperative problems.

Urodynamics, in combination with a thorough urological history and physical examination, forms the cornerstone of the evaluation of these more complex patients.

## PATIENT EVALUATION

Incontinence carries considerable social stigma that recently has only lessened due to an increased awareness of the problem, but many sufferers are still reluctant to seek advice or treatment. Some patients are able to overcome incontinence by passing urine frequently or restricting their fluid intake and physical activities that may cause the problem. Others cope with incontinence by wearing pads or other devices.

All patients who have incontinence should be encouraged to seek expert medical advice because most cases are amenable to some form of therapy to improve their symptoms.

A careful medical history should be taken with particular emphasis on:
- factors that induce leakage;
- obstetric history;
- surgical history; and
- drug therapy.

Clinical examination may reveal palpable enlargement of the bladder or stress leakage with or without prolapse when the patient coughs.

Urodynamic evaluation is important in the assessment of all forms of incontinence, but may not be necessary for straightforward cases of stress incontinence.

An algorithm for the investigation of incontinence is shown in Figure 5.1.

Initially it is most important to differentiate incontinence due to detrusor overactivity from incontinence due to inadequate outflow resistance, although these conditions can coexist.

### Definition of the overactive bladder

There is a complex of symptoms associated with the bladder overactivity seen with detrusor instability and hyperreflexia. This clinical grouping has been named the overactive bladder and includes the symptoms of frequency, urgency and/or urge incontinence. Frequency is partly a result of a low functional bladder capacity, but can also partly be a result of an adaptive or coping mechanism to suppress urgency. The overactive bladder can be defined as the clinical condition characterized by the symptoms of frequency, urgency and/or urge incontinence occurring in the absence of any identifiable local pathology. Inherent in this diagnosis is the fact that these symptoms may also be caused by other bladder disorders that might require treatment; therefore accurate investigation to exclude other significant pathology is essential for the effective management of these patients who have an overactive bladder.

In the absence of other identifiable pathology it is thought that these irritative symptoms are caused by uncontrolled contractions of the detrusor while the bladder is filling with urine and therefore result from detrusor

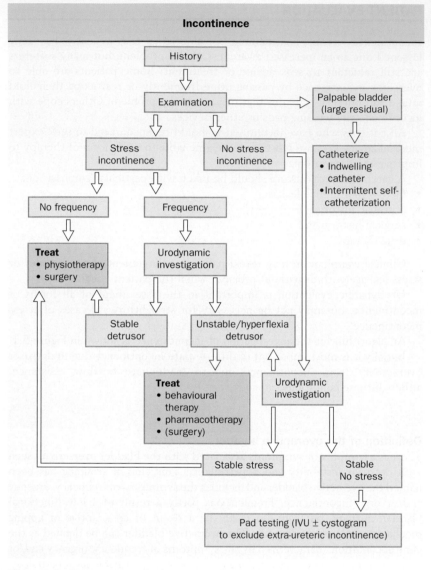

**Figure 5.1  Management of urinary incontinence.** (IVU, intravenous urogram.)
Particular indications for urodynamics.

- failed empirical therapy;
- mixed stress/urge incontinence:
- raised residual urine volume;
- previous failed surgery;
- history of neurological disease.

**100**

instability. Although it is clear that the diagnosis of detrusor instability and detrusor hyperreflexia can only be made on the basis of a urodynamic study, there is a place for a presumptive clinical diagnosis that may equate with detrusor instability and detrusor hyperreflexia in routine clinical practice outside specialist centres (Figure 5.2).

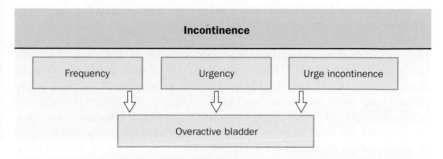

**Figure 5.2  Symptoms of overactive bladder.**

Any clinician making a diagnosis of overactive bladder must ensure that other significant pathology is excluded and that this diagnosis is only considered after the judicious use of routine clinical investigations (e.g. midstream urine examination). Overactive bladder may be due to a number of causes which include:

- idiopathic;
- behavioural;
- bladder outlet obstruction;
- anatomic (pelvic floor/urethral disorder);
- intravesical;
- myogenic; and
- neurogenic.

The symptom complex of overactive bladder is troublesome and forms one of the most common health problems affecting both men and women of all ages. Most studies reporting the prevalence of this condition have focused on urinary leakage (urge incontinence), which is only one of the symptoms and occurs in only about one-third of cases of overactive bladder. Approximately 70% of people with overactive bladder suffer from frequency and urgency symptoms that can also severely disrupt their daily lifestyle. The real extent of overactive bladder has therefore been seriously underestimated. Recent work reviewing 17000 people in six European countries suggests that the prevalence of overactive bladder is 12–22% of all people aged 40 years or over. In the USA it has been estimated that at least 17 million people suffer from overactive bladder.

The cause of overactive bladder is usually unknown, but it can be treated by inhibiting bladder contraction with antimuscarinic drugs, either alone or in combination with bladder training. Successful management of patients who have overactive bladder requires that the condition is accurately diagnosed and differentiated from other bladder problems such as stress incontinence.

An overactive bladder can have a profound effect on the daily activities of those who have it. Despite its prevalence, many people with overactive bladder do not seek medical attention for a variety of reasons such as being too embarrassed to consult a medical practitioner to believing that their condition is 'inevitable'. Others are unaware of the treatment options available or have not benefited from previous treatment. As a result many people who have an overactive bladder endure the inconvenience and unpleasantness of their symptoms of frequency, urgency and urge incontinence for many years, often developing elaborate coping mechanisms to manage their condition. The coping mechanisms may include voiding frequently, mapping out the location of toilets, drinking less or wearing dark clothing to mask incontinent episodes. Others resort to wearing incontinence pads or sanitary towels to cope with the urge incontinence.

Many different types of problems – social, psychological, occupational, domestic, physical and sexual – have been identified among people who have an overactive bladder. These include reduced social interaction, depression,

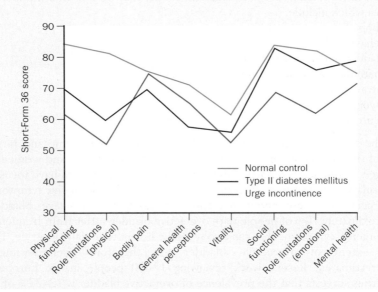

**Figure 5.3   Effects of overactive bladder and type II diabetes mellitus on the quality of life domains of the Short-Form 36 quality of life questionnaire.**

disrupted sleep patterns, absence from work and avoidance of physical activities. The quality of life of those who have an overactive bladder has recently been compared with that of the 'normal' population using the Short-Form 36 (SF36) questionnaire – a widely used generic method for quantifying quality of life. Overall quality of life was significantly impaired (p<0.0001) in six of the eight domains of the SF36 for people who had an overactive bladder when compared with individuals of a similar age and sex in the general population. In addition, overactive bladder was found to have a greater negative impact on quality of life than type II diabetes mellitus (Figure 5.3). This was particularly true for the emotional domains, which include social functioning and emotional role limitations.

The effects of a disease on quality of life can also be evaluated by the amount that patients are willing to pay, in addition to any reimbursed cost, for effective and side-effect-free alleviation of their symptoms. Many people who have an overactive bladder have a strong desire for effective and well-tolerated treatment, evidenced by the high value that they are willing to pay, in addition to the real costs of health care, that they place on such treatment (Figure 5.4). This clearly indicates that overactive bladder has a substantial adverse effect on quality of life.

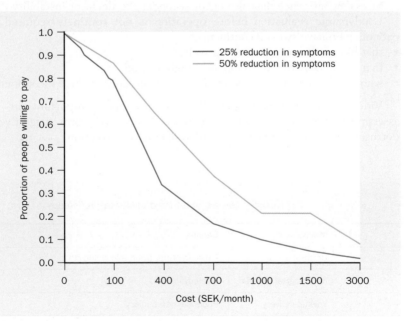

**Figure 5.4  Proportion of people who have overactive bladder or mixed incontinence willing to pay defined amounts for a new side-effect-free treatment.** 1 US$ ~ 7.7 Swedish krona (SEK). (Reproduced with permission from Johannesson *et al.* British Journal of Urology 1997;80:557–562.)

## GENUINE STRESS INCONTINENCE

### Definition

Genuine stress incontinence (GSI) is defined as incontinence associated with activities such as coughing, sneezing, running, and jumping that increase intra-abdominal pressure and also the intravesical pressure leading to urine leakage.

GSI is predominantly a female problem and is particularly common in multiparous women who have had traumatic or prolonged vaginal deliveries (Figure 5.5). It is due to reduced outflow resistance which may be at the level of:

- the bladder neck;
- the striated urethral sphincter; or
- both the bladder neck and the striated urethral sphincter.

There is some dispute about the relative importance of bladder base prolapse, opening of the bladder neck, and striated sphincter integrity in the aetiology of GSI. It is likely that all patients who have GSI have some degree of intrinsic sphincter deficiency (Figure 5.6). The elderly may have other irritative symptoms as a result of tissue atrophy and oestrogen deficiency.

Stress incontinence may also occur secondary to detrusor instability.

Urodynamic evaluation before operation is not routinely required for patients who have stress incontinence:

- that has not been treated operatively;
- that is clinically demonstrable on coughing; and
- who do not complain of urinary frequency, urgency, or urge incontinence.

Videocystometrography (VCMG) is, however, important in the assessment of stress incontinence associated with symptoms suggestive of detrusor instability or a history of failed operative correction.

| Contributory causes to intrinsic sphincter deficiency | |
|---|---|
| **Mechanism** | **Causes** |
| Urethral trauma | Pelvic fracture, traumatic childbirth |
| Neurological disorder | Myelodysplasia |
| Vaginal delivery | Pudendal nerve injury |
| Previous operation | Failed operation for incontinence, urethral dilatation, urethral diverticulectomy, radical prostatectomy |

Figure 5.5   Contributory causes to intrinsic sphincter deficiency.

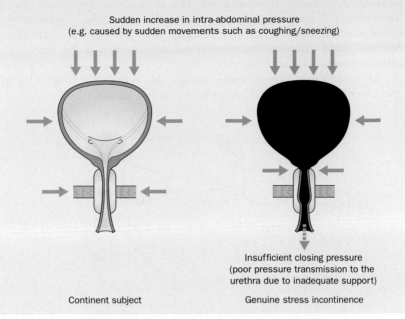

Figure 5.6   Mechanism of genuine stress incontinence.

## History and examination

Important factors in the history are:
* actions that induce stress incontinence; and
* an assessment of the amount leaked.

Associated frequency, urgency, and urge incontinence suggest the possibility of stress incontinence in association with detrusor instability.

Examination may reveal:
* anterior or posterior vaginal wall prolapse;
* introital atrophy; or
* urethral mucosal prolapse.

These findings may be of significance in the aetiology.

The patient should be asked to cough and perform a Valsalva manoeuvre in both the lying and standing or squatting positions. The degree of prolapse of the vaginal walls and cervix should be examined and the presence and amount of stress incontinence observed. It is preferable to perform the examination when the patient has a full bladder. It is best to assess prolapse with the patient lying in the left lateral position. Assessment of the degree of bladder base and urethral prolapse is difficult because of the subjectivity involved. An attempt to standardize this subject has been made by the International Continence Society (Figure 5.7), but the classification is complex and is likely to remain a research tool. The most accurate way of defining the anatomical and functional abnormality is by the use of videocystometry (Figure 5.8).

If sphincteric incontinence occurs in association with detrusor overactivity so-called 'mixed incontinence' is said to occur.

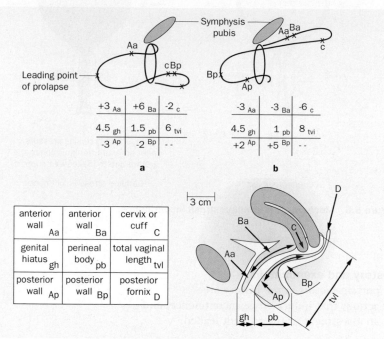

**Figure 5.7   Grid and line diagrams for documenting uterine prolapse. (a) Stage III-Ba prolapse. (b) Stage III-Bp prolapse.** (Reproduced with permission ICS Standardisation; Bump RC, et al. The standardization of terminology of female pelvic organ prolapse and pelvic floor dysfunction. American Journal of Obstetrics and Gynecology 1996; 175:10–17.) Valsalva leak point pressures (VLPP) are commonly used in some areas of the world. Low pressures (<60 cm $H_2O$) have been suggested to equate with intrinsic sphincter deficiency, but the evidence in support of this is contradictory (p. 47). There is debate over the 'ideal' conditions for the VLPP test and recent work has suggested that the VLPP test is only positive in two-thirds of cases who demonstrate leakage on being asked to cough.

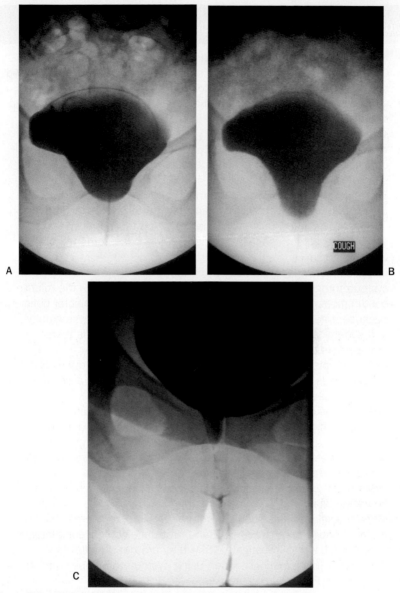

A

B

C

Figure 5.8    (A) Cystogram with patient in the supine position showing a degree of bladder base prolapse. (B) The same patient on coughing showing descent of the bladder base and urethra, on the dynamic screening image leaking was visible. (C) Cystourethrogram showing typical patient with intrinsic sphincter deficiency with a well supported bladder base and contrast on coughing filling the urethra with associated leakage.

## URODYNAMICS IN PRACTICE: GENUINE STRESS INCONTINENCE

- No postmicturition residual urine (Figure 5.9)
- Cystometry is not necessary for clinically demonstrable uncomplicated stress incontinence without symptoms of detrusor instability
- Indications for urodynamic evaluation are the possibility of associated detrusor instability and a previous history of failure to respond to a surgical operation
- With videourodynamics (VCMG), fluoroscopy during filling may reveal opening of the bladder neck and descent of the bladder base in the supine or standing positions
- There is no consensus about the most appropriate definition for the presence of intrinsic sphincter deficiency – alternatives include history (at least 20% inaccuracy), examination (Q tip test), urodynamics, urethral pressure measurements, leak point measurements, and videourodynamics
- In our opinion videocystometry or certainly the use of cystourethrography is essential to allow differentiation of the relative contributions of bladder base prolapse and intrinsic sphincter deficiency because it deals with function (cystometry), anatomy (cystography), and dynamics (screening) – is the bladder neck open? is there prolapse? is there demonstrable leakage?
- In GSI the pressure should not rise above the baseline during filling – cough leak is almost always demonstrable and is often associated with bladder base descent
- Voiding is usually rapid and complete with a high flow rate (30–60 ml/s) and low voiding pressure due to reduced outflow resistance
- Many patients are unable to interrupt micturition due to weakness of their striated sphincter mechanism
- The amount of urinary leakage the patient experiences in daily life may be assessed by pad weighing (see pp. 23–26)
- More specialized tests such as urethral profilometry (see pp. 60–63), the fluid bridge test (see p. 60), and urethral electrical conductance have been used to investigate GSI – they are not beneficial in diagnosis in our experience when using cystourethrography and should be reserved for research purposes
- Endoscopy probably adds little to the evaluation of patients who have anatomical stress incontinence, but is helpful in assessing the short fibrotic 'stove-pipe' urethra sometimes present in patients who have intrinsic sphincter deficiency. Complex patients suspected of having a bladder fistula or urethral diverticulum require diagnostic endoscopy

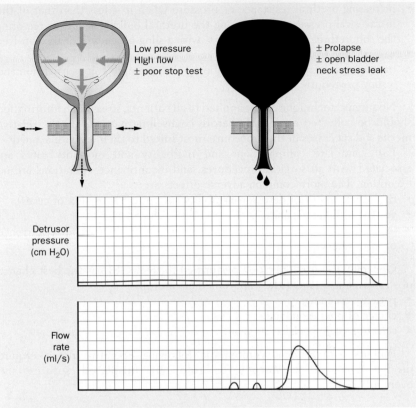

Low pressure
High flow
± poor stop test

± Prolapse
± open bladder
neck stress leak

Detrusor
pressure
(cm H₂O)

Flow
rate
(ml/s)

**Figure 5.9  Typical cystometrogram and videocystometrogram appearances for genuine stress incontinence.**

## Management

Treatment of GSI is aimed at correcting prolapse and increasing outflow resistance. Conservative treatments include:
- pelvic floor exercises;
- cones;
- electrical stimulation;  and
- incontinence devices such as the Fem Assist™ and Reliance™ urethral plugs.

These treatments are useful alternatives to a surgical operation, which may be inappropriate. However, operative treatment is more effective and aims include:
- elevating the bladder neck to a position where intra-abdominal pressure transmission to this region is identical to that transmitted to the bladder (e.g. Burch colposuspension);

- increasing urethral resistance or pressure when it is less than that of the intravesical pressure at rest, using the urethral bulking agents or restoring the suburethral 'hammock support' with a sling procedure or tension-free vaginal tape technique;
- producing a combination of the above – for example colposuspension and a sling procedure.

No surgical technique can be applied to all patients, so as much information should be collected as possible before counselling patients on the relative merits and successes of the procedure most suited to their individual needs.

Early and late complications and morbidity and mortality rates are associated with all surgical procedures, and incontinence operations are no exception. The more common adverse effects are:
- the development of detrusor instability (in up to 5% to 10% of cases);
- voiding difficulties; and
- less often, immediate failure of the operative technique or late recurrence of incontinence.

Generally the first operation performed to treat GSI has the best chance of success, emphasizing the importance of careful:
- patient screening;
- choice of operation; and
- selection of a specialist surgeon.

Patients who remain symptomatic following operative repair require urodynamics and cystoscopy to rule out misplaced sutures and overcorrection.

## PRIMARY DETRUSOR INSTABILITY

The normal bladder is compliant and detrusor pressure should not increase during filling unless overfilled to the point where the overfilling causes discomfort.

Detrusor instability or the unstable bladder describes a bladder that is objectively shown to contract spontaneously or on provocation during the filling or storage phase of cystometry while the patient is attempting to inhibit micturition (Figure 5.10). There is an involuntary increase in detrusor pressure when the patient is not attempting to void and this can cause symptoms of urgency and urge incontinence (Figure 5.11).

When such an increase in detrusor pressure is associated with a known neurological deficit the alternative term of detrusor hyperreflexia should be used. It is important to appreciate the association between the overactive bladder, the urodynamic diagnosis of detrusor instability or hyperreflexia and other potential bladder pathology (e.g. carcinoma *in situ* or sensory bladder disorder; Figure 5.12).

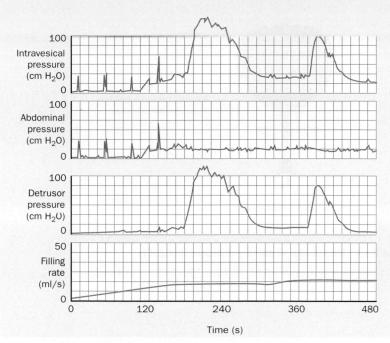

**Figure 5.10  Primary detrusor instability.**

There are two main patterns of detrusor overactivity:
- phasic or systolic – the pressure increases are in a wave form; and
- hypocompliant – the pressure increase is linearly related to the filled volume.

On occasions there may be combined hypocompliance and phasic contractions (see below).

Detrusor instability may develop secondary to bladder outflow obstruction, most commonly in elderly men who have benign prostatic hyperplasia, but also in:
- boys who have urethral valves;
- young males who have bladder neck dyssynergia; and
- females after operative treatment for stress incontinence.

Idiopathic or primary detrusor instability is defined as detrusor instability that is not secondary to outflow obstruction. Its aetiology is not fully understood, but it may be triggered in certain individuals by coughing, giggling (particularly in young girls), or female orgasm.

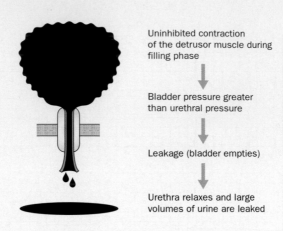

Uninhibited contraction
of the detrusor muscle during
filling phase

↓

Bladder pressure greater
than urethral pressure

↓

Leakage (bladder empties)

↓

Urethra relaxes and large
volumes of urine are leaked

Figure 5.11    Mechanism of primary detrusor instability.

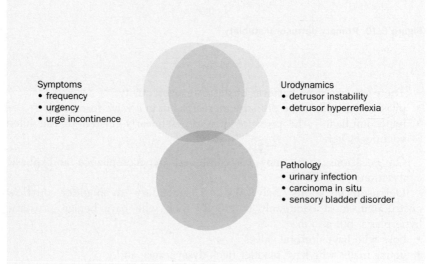

Symptoms
• frequency
• urgency
• urge incontinence

Urodynamics
• detrusor instability
• detrusor hyperreflexia

Pathology
• urinary infection
• carcinoma in situ
• sensory bladder disorder

Figure 5.12    Symptoms of overactive bladder.

## History and examination

Patients who have detrusor instability may complain of frequency and urgency and if severe, urge incontinence. They may also have stress incontinence secondary to opening of the bladder neck due to an increase in the intravesical pressure. Other presentations of hyperactive detrusor functions include:

- unconscious incontinence;
- flooding incontinence;
- giggle incontinence;
- incontinence during intercourse;
- adult enuresis;
- 'obstructed' voiding pattern;
- double voiding; and
- typical triggers: running water, key in the door syndrome, foot on the floor syndrome.

Examination is usually unremarkable, but it is important to check that the bladder is not palpable (suggesting retention with overflow incontinence). Neurological examination might reveal a deficit suggesting detrusor hyperreflexia. It is therefore important to check that:

- sensation in the sacral dermatomes is not impaired;
- there is no muscle wasting;
- there is no weakness or disturbance of reflexes in the lower limbs;
- anal sphincter tone is not decreased.

### URODYNAMICS IN PRACTICE: PRIMARY DETRUSOR INSTABILITY

- Free flow rate is characteristically high
- Time to maximum flow is reduced (often <2 s)
- On initial catheterization it is unusual to find any residual urine
- During filling, the pressure increases above baseline in a physiological fashion and at this point the patient usually complains of urgency and impending incontinence
- The pattern of unstable detrusor contractions is usually phasic or systolic in appearance (Figure 5.14), but on occasion there is a linear rise referred to as hypocompliance
- Hypocompliance may result from fibrosis of the bladder wall (the so-called plastic bag effect) but also occurs in the neuropathic bladder
- Overstretching of the normal bladder to the point where the subject experiences severe pain may induce a hypocompliant pressure rise and this should be avoided
- On occasions a mixed picture can be seen and systolic pressure waves may be superimposed upon a hypocompliant pressure rise

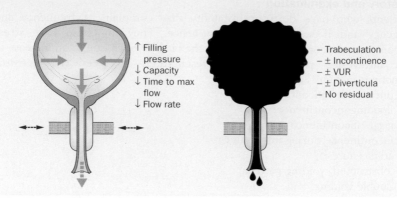

**Figure 5.13   Typical cystometrogram and videocystometrogram appearances for primary detrusor instability (or hyperreflexia).** VUR, vesicoureteral reflux.

- Fluoroscopy of the unstable bladder during filling usually demonstrates trabeculation of the bladder and occasionally diverticula
- Opening of the bladder neck may be seen associated with pressure rises, particularly in females, and this may lead to secondary stress incontinence
- Vesicoureteral reflux is more common in association with high detrusor pressures and may be seen on fluoroscopy
- Voiding is usually rapid and with a high flow rate and normal voiding pressure
- A stop test is not always possible due to the force of the detrusor contraction, but when successful the isometric pressure contraction ($p$Iso) is often high (>50 cm $H_2O$)
- Usually void to completion, but associated diverticula may not empty
- Vesicoureteral reflux may occur during voiding, particularly at the time of the stop test when the intravesical pressure is elevated

## Management
### *Exclude an intravesical lesion (Fig. 5.15)*
Cystourethroscopy is useful to exclude calculi and tumours if symptoms dictate or pharmacological treatments fail to improve symptoms.

### *Bladder training – behavioural therapy*
Having excluded an irritative lesion the next therapeutic approach is bladder training – the patient is instructed to make a conscious effort to resist the desire to void and to void only when the bladder feels absolutely full. Such

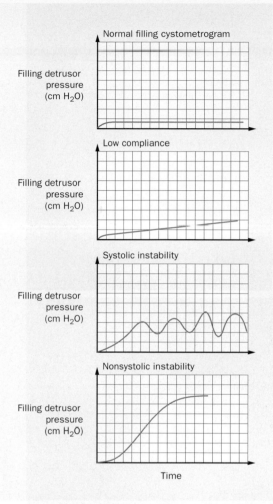

**Figure 5.14   Cystometrogram patterns of filling detrusor pressure.**

training can be assisted by supplying patients with 'time and amount' or 'frequency–volume' charts because by careful analysis of their micturition pattern they may acquire greater insight so helping to resolve the problem. This can be accompanied by advice on simple measures such as:

- timed voiding
- decreasing excessive fluid intake;
- avoiding tea, coffee, and alcohol; or
- changing drinking habits.

**115**

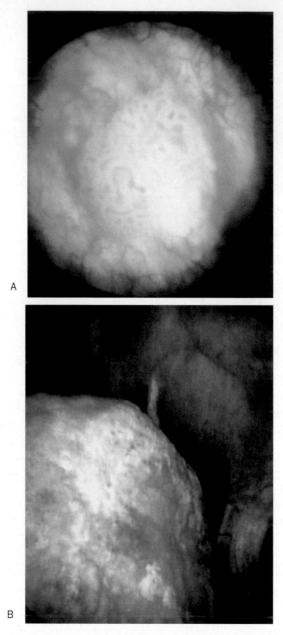

Figure 5.15 (A) A superficial transitional cell carcinoma of the bladder in a patient with irritative voiding symptoms. (B) Cystoscopic evidence of a stitch and bladder calculus in a patient with irritative symptoms following an abdominal hysterectomy.

*Drug therapy*

Drug therapy is either used primarily in conjunction with bladder training, or following a failure of bladder training. The mechanism of action of the majority of current agents used to treat detrusor instability relies upon their anticholinergic antimuscarinic properties. The management is directed towards:

- inhibiting unstable bladder contractions;
- increasing bladder compliance; and
- decreasing sensory input to increase bladder capacity and decrease symptoms.

The main agents available are reviewed in Figure 5.16 derived from the recent World Health Organization report, but the principal agents in use are:
- tolterodine 2 mg twice daily except in hepatically impaired patients (in these patients 1 mg bd)
- immediate release oxybutynin 2.5–5 mg three times a day or extended release oxybutynin 5–30 mg od.

Side effects such as dryness of the mouth and dizziness are particularly commonly encountered with oxybutynin and some patients are unable to tolerate these side effects in long-term use – in fact less than 20% will remain on therapy. Tolterodine has a lower incidence of side effects.

The tricyclic antidepressant imipramine (25–100 mg at bedtime) is particularly useful for elderly patients who have nocturia because in addition to its anticholinergic effect it also has a sedative action.

Desmopressin is a synthetic analogue of vasopressin. This antidiuretic agent, given intranasally in a dose of 20–40 µg before going to bed, reduces nocturnal urine production by up to 50%; it is now also available as an oral formulation, 200–400 µg nocte. It is useful for treating nocturia and bedwetting. Caution is needed when it is used by elderly patients because of the potentially serious incidence of fluid retention and subsequent cardiac compromise.

There is considerable interest and several ongoing clinical trials are underway to find other effective pharmacological agents with more acceptable side effect profiles. Other agents include propiverine and trospium chloride and new routes and formulations for oxybutynin are being explored.

If drug therapy fails to control the symptoms or causes intolerable side effects operative intervention should be considered.

There has been a vogue for subtrigonal injection of phenol in female patients, but this has been abandoned due to unacceptable side effects such as fistula formation, sciatic nerve damage, and ureteric fibrosis. In particular this technique should be avoided in the male because it often leads to impotence. Bladder distension was popular in the 1970s but has no benefit except in the treatment of interstitial cystitis.

**Available pharmacotherapy for bladder overactivity**

| Drugs | Pharmacological and/or physiological evidence | Clinical evidence | Assessment |
|---|---|---|---|
| *Antimuscarinic* | | | |
| Atropine, hyoscyamine | E | C | - |
| Propantheline | E | A | R |
| Emepronium | E | A/B | R |
| Trospium | E | A | R |
| Tolterodine | E | A | R |
| (Darifenacin) | | Under investigation | |
| *Drugs acting on membrane channels* | | | |
| Calcium antagonists | | Under investigation | |
| Potassium channel openers | | Under investigation | |
| *Drugs with mixed actions* | | | |
| Oxybutynin | E | A | R |
| Dicyclomine | E | B | - |
| Propiverine | E | A | R |
| Flavoxate | U | B/C | - |
| *Alpha adrenoceptor antagonists* | | | |
| Alfuzosin | U | B/C | - |
| Doxazosin | U | B/C | - |
| Prazosin | U | B/C | - |
| Terazosin | U | B/C | - |
| Tamusulosin | U | B/C | - |
| *Beta adrenoceptor antagonists* | | | |
| Terbutaline | U | B/C | - |
| Clenbuterol | U | B/C | - |
| Salbutamol | U | C | - |
| *Antidepressants* | | | |
| Imipramine | E | A | R |
| *Prostaglandin synthesis inhibitors* | | | |
| Indomethacin | U | B | - |
| Flurbiprofen | U | B | - |

Figure 5.16   Drugs used to treat detrusor instability.

**Available pharmacotherapy for bladder overactivity**

| Drugs | Pharmacological and/or physiological evidence | Clinical evidence | Assessment |
|---|---|---|---|
| *Vasopressin analogues* Desmopressin | E | A | R |
| *Other drugs* Baclofen Capsaicin Resiniferatoxin | E E | C B Under investigation | - - |

E = efficacious; U = unproven; A = good quality RCT; B = clinical studies;
C = expert opinion, R = recommended.
With permission of WHO Consultation on Incontinence 1998.

**Figure 5.16** (contd)

Our favoured operative treatment for intractable detrusor instability is the 'clam' enterocystoplasty. The bladder is divided through a suprapubic incision in the coronal or sagittal direction down to the trigone, taking care to preserve the ureters. A measured segment of terminal ileum and its mesentery are resected and the bowel is opened along its antimesenteric border. The patch of bowel is then sutured to the free edges of the divided bladder. Patients undergoing this operation are warned of the potential necessity for intermittent clean self-catheterization if the augmented bladder fails to empty satisfactorily.

Less invasive alternatives are being investigated, for example:

- autoaugmentation, which involves the production of a pseudodiverticulum on the bladder; and
- neuromodulation, which involves extradural stimulation of the third sacral nerve root.

Approximately 30% of patients may benefit from neuromodulation. Although it represents a minimally invasive alternative for these patients, the implants are, however, extremely costly. The exact mechanism of sacral nerve stimulation is not clear, but it is believed that the stimulation of A$\delta$ myelinated fibres, especially at the S3 level, enhances sphincter and pelvic tone and may result in an inhibitory effect on the detrusor reflex. A temporary stimulating wire is inserted first to assess the method before a permanent implant is placed.

## CYSTOPLASTY URODYNAMICS

Enterocystoplasty using small or large bowel has become increasingly popular as a treatment for bladder dysfunction. All patients for whom such a procedure is planned should undergo careful urodynamic evaluation before the operation. 'Clam' cystoplasty using a segment of terminal ileum is now popular as a treatment for detrusor hyperreflexia and primary detrusor instability.

Substitution cystoplasty using caecum, colon, or a pouch constructed from segments of ileum is a useful technique for increasing bladder capacity in cases where the capacity is restricted due to interstitial cystitis, postirradiation fibrosis, or tuberculous contracture. In addition some cases of bladder carcinoma are suitable for subtotal cystectomy and cystoplasty using similar techniques. Cystoplasty can be performed using intact segments of bowel, detubularized bowel (in which the tubular structure is surgically altered), or pouches.

Following cystoplasty some patients experience persistent or new symptoms such as urinary frequency and incontinence, voiding difficulty, or recurrent urinary tract infections. Videocystometrography is important in the evaluation of such cases. Bowel segment peristalsis is usually as it would be in its usual situation. Voiding is achieved by abdominal straining, which is more efficient when coincident with peristaltic contractions. High-pressure peristaltic contractions can lead to urinary frequency, urgency, and incontinence. This is a rare occurrence, but more likely when non-detubularized bowel segments are used.

Videocystometrography is particularly useful in the assessment of complicated postcystoplasty cases and attention can be paid to several important factors:
- is the cystoplasty overactive?
- is this overactivity associated with outflow obstruction?
- is incontinence due to hyperactivity of the bowel segment or impaired outflow resistance?

The presence or absence of postmicturition residual urine is better assessed by ultrasound cystodynamogram, but videocystometrography may clarify the aetiology.

### Management
Overactive cystoplasties associated with outflow obstruction are best treated by first relieving the obstruction:
- in females this usually means urethral dilatation; and
- in males bladder neck incision or transurethral prostatectomy may be indicated.

Mucus production by the bowel segment can lead to the formation of mucus plugs that can cause intermittent obstruction. It has recently been shown that a regular intake of cranberry juice can lead to decreased mucus production and so prevent such obstruction.

Hyperactive cystoplasties without obstruction are best treated by pharmacotherapy initially. Anticholinergic therapy such as oxybutynin or tolterodine is usually used. In the authors' experience these agents are not generally helpful in treating hyperactive cystoplasties. Also drugs such as mebeverine that are administered orally as a treatment for irritable colon are not sufficiently well absorbed to act upon bowel segments separated from the alimentary tract and are therefore not effective for hyperactive cystoplasties.

If drug therapy fails and the symptoms resulting from overactivity of the cystoplasty are sufficiently severe then a further operation – detubularization – is indicated. It is often most convenient to add a patch of small bowel to the side of the cystoplasty using the same concept as the 'clam' cystoplasty.

Underactivity or absent peristalsis in cystoplasties is more likely to occur after detubularization of the bowel segment. Many patients, particularly females, are able to void to completion by abdominal straining and so experience no adverse symptoms. However, underactive cystoplasties can be associated with a large postmicturition residual urine volume, which in turn can lead to recurrent urinary tract infections. This problem is more likely to occur in males, in whom outflow resistance is higher and so abdominal straining is less efficient. When large residual volumes are associated with recurrent infections, intermittent self-catheterization is often indicated and can be helpful in relieving such problems.

# Chapter 6 | Sensory disorders

## INTRODUCTION

Urodynamic investigations were originally developed to study the 'motor' function of the lower urinary tract, but some information can also be acquired on bladder sensation. Indeed it has been recognised in recent years that the sensory arc of the voiding reflex is important in determining voiding function and may play a role in the aetiology of detrusor instability.

Bladder sensation can be assessed using stimulating electrodes introduced through the urethra, but such techniques are used for research purposes rather than routine assessment. Urodynamic tests are not ideal techniques for evaluating sensory disorders, but enable the observer to:
- measure the sensory threshold objectively; and
- exclude motor disorders.

Abnormalities of bladder sensation can be broadly categorized into hypersensitive and hyposensitive disorders.

## HYPERSENSITIVITY OF THE LOWER URINARY TRACT

### Causes
Hypersensitivity of the lower urinary tract may be idiopathic, but is often due to inflammation within the bladder or urethra. Causes include:
- bacterial cystitis (the commonest cause) – it is important to ensure that there is no concurrent infection during urodynamics because the test will often exacerbate the urinary infection, which may lead to a bacteraemia and cannot usually be interpreted due to the inflammation-induced 'hypersensitivity';
- other infective processes include human papillomavirus infection within the urethra and trigone in females and urethritis and chronic prostatitis in males; and
- other inflammatory conditions such as bladder calculus, bladder carcinoma, postradiation cystitis, cyclophosphamide cystitis, chemical cystitis, and interstitial cystitis.

There is also a group of patients in whom hypersensitivity exists without evidence of inflammation of the bladder, but where instrumentation of the urethra is extremely painful. This condition is sometimes referred to as urethral syndrome. It usually occurs in young women and may respond to urethral dilatation.

## Hypersensitive bladder

A hypersensitive bladder is defined as a disorder leading to increased urinary frequency, which may be accompanied by urgency and bladder pain, in which cystometry fails to demonstrate a rise in the filling detrusor pressure above baseline. A management plan for the hypersensitive bladder is shown in Figure 6.1.

### History and examination

A full history is particularly important in the assessment of hypersensitive disorders of the bladder. Clinical features can include:

- urinary frequency – a prominent symptom for which bladder pain rather than impending incontinence is the trigger;
- urgency, but incontinence is uncommon;
- daytime frequency;
- bladder pain – usually relieved by voiding, but with many factors suggestive of bacterial cystitis and a negative mid-stream urine;
- dysuria;
- dyspareunia – a common symptom;
- strangury – suggestive of trigonal inflammation; and
- occasionally haematuria, which requires investigation of both the bladder and upper tracts.

The symptoms are chronic. Typically there is a previous probable urinary tract infection, but often a urine culture has not been performed. The patient receives a course of antibiotics and the symptoms disappear for a while. However, urine cultures reveal that the urine is sterile, antibiotics do not improve the condition, and the symptoms persist. Women often report improvement at the end of their menstrual cycle and many will have had previous hysterectomy, perhaps for lower abdominal pain, but no obvious gynaecological pathology.

Examination may be unremarkable, but attention should be paid to the urethral meatus, which may be inflamed or show mucosal prolapse (a urethral caruncle). There may also be bladder tenderness, both suprapubically and on vaginal examination. A gentle bimanual examination will identify other pelvic pathology.

All cases require urinalysis and culture; urine cytology is recommended for selected cases (see Figure 6.1). Radiography is generally not useful, but pelvic ultrasound may be helpful in excluding gynaecological disease.

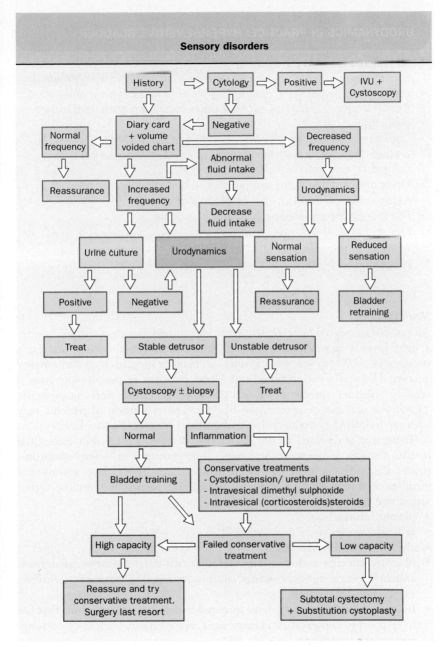

**Figure 6.1 Management of hypersensitive bladder disorders.**

**URODYNAMICS IN PRACTICE: HYPERSENSITIVE BLADDER**

- All patients who have symptoms suggestive of a hypersensitive bladder should have urine culture and if negative a urodynamic assessment
- Urodynamics is helpful in diagnosing patients who have hypersensitive painful bladders and helps exclude other conditions such as detrusor overactivity
- Catheterization may be painful – passage of the catheter through the urethra and contact with the bladder mucosa may cause pain suggesting the urethral syndrome
- Major diagnostic features are premature first sensation of filling and reduced bladder capacity due to bladder discomfort
- Filling pressure and voiding function are normal
- The diagnosis of a 'hypersensitive bladder' is one of exclusion and relies upon the exclusion of other intravesical pathology including malignancy

## Management

All cases of suspected hypersensitive bladder should have a cystoscopy under a light general anaesthesia combined with bladder hydrodistension (at a pressure of >100 cm water for 5 min) and bladder biopsies if an abnormality is seen. There is a rise in pulse and blood pressure in people who have a sensory bladder problem. Postdistension bleeding and nonspecific 'glomerulations' can be seen in the bladder. The symptoms of patients may improve following cystodistension and urethral recalibration to 42 F.

Treatment is directed at the underlying disease process, but interstitial cystitis remains of unknown aetiology. Those patients in whom symptoms persist despite treatment may gain symptomatic relief from intravesical instillation of dimethyl sulphoxide, heparinoid agents or steroids. Other supportive treatments include:

- patient information;
- self-help groups (local and national);
- alterations in diet and fluids;
- pharmacotherapy including non-steroidal anti-inflammatories, analgesics, anticholinergics, antidepressants, antihistamines, $H_2$ antagonists, elmiron and corticosteroids; and
- for those few patients who have intractable debilitating symptoms that fail to respond to conservative management, open surgery such as cystectomy and enterocystoplasty.

Treatment of bladder hypersensitivity due to infection or mucosal inflammation is beyond the scope of this book.

## IMPAIRED BLADDER SENSATION OR 'HYPOSENSITIVE BLADDER'

Hyposensitive bladder is defined as impaired bladder sensation leading to loss or reduction of the desire to micturate and therefore infrequent micturition and a large capacity bladder. In its early stages this is purely a sensory problem that may lead to detrusor underactivity and insufficient bladder emptying. In the long term there is detrusor failure due to chronic overdistension of the bladder.

Hyposensitive bladder is usually due to denervation. Causes include:

- spinal cord injury (the best known cause) in which the sensory pathways are interrupted;
- pelvic trauma and radical surgery such as Wertheim's radical hysterectomy and abdominoperineal resection of the rectum (may lead to impairment of bladder sensation due to local denervation).

There is also a group of predominantly female patients in whom the desire to micturate when the bladder is full is impaired for no apparent reason. These people void infrequently and have a large capacity bladder without evidence of obstruction or detrusor dysfunction and the condition is sometimes referred to as 'camel bladder'.

### History and examination

Patients who have a hyposensitive bladder may have no symptoms apart from loss of the desire to micturate. Other symptoms can include:

- recurrent urinary tract infection;
- urinary frequency and incontinence secondary to poor bladder emptying;
- straining to urinate with a poor flow; and
- a feeling of incomplete emptying.

The patient may have a previous history of spinal cord or cauda equina injury or pelvic surgery causing bladder denervation.

A number of acquired peripheral neuropathies, the most common being diabetic autonomic neuropathy, may affect the peripheral innervation of the bladder, predominantly the sensory nerve endings.

Some individuals give a history of chronic urine holding resulting in overdistension of the bladder muscle and myogenic failure.

It is unusual for post-trauma cases to have a selective sensory problem, most being combined with detrusor underactivity. Examination may reveal impaired sensation on testing sensation in sacral dermatomes.

## URODYNAMICS IN PRACTICE: HYPOSENSITIVE BLADDER

- The characteristic urodynamic features are an increase in the volume at which the first sensation of filling occurs and a high maximum cystometric capacity
- In severe cases there may be almost no bladder sensation and voiding needs to be initiated without any desire to micturate 'by the clock'
- In pure hyposensitivity detrusor function during filling and voiding is normal
- Detrusor failure results in the inability to generate a detrusor contraction and a high postvoid residual urine volume

### Management

The treatment of bladder hyposensitivity is bladder training – the patient is encouraged to void 'by the clock' about six times a day and double void even though the desire to void may be absent. If such treatment is started early in the course of the condition it should prevent subsequent futher impairment of detrusor function. Ultimately clean intermittent self-catheterization is the best treatment for those who have symptomatic inefficient bladder emptying and urinary retention. It is important to monitor these patients carefully particularly if they are not using ISC to check that they do not develop 'chronic retention' with increasing residuals.

# Chapter 7 | The contracted bladder

The contracted bladder is defined as a reduction in the functional capacity of the bladder due to fibrotic contracture or carcinoma within the bladder wall.

Causes of fibrotic contracture include:

- previous irradiation;
- tuberculosis;
- chemical cystitis;
- interstitial cystitis; and
- schistosomiasis.

Fibrotic contracture is preceded by inflammation so hypersensitivity and contracture may coexist. However, the final stage of the condition may not be accompanied by hypersensitivity.

## History and examination

The patient will usually have a previous long history of an aetiological factor listed above. Symptoms can include:

- urinary frequency by day and night – usually the predominant complaint;
- urgency – often present;
- stress incontinence – often present; and
- bladder pain on filling if there is concurrent inflammation of the bladder.

Examination is usually unremarkable although there may be some suprapubic tenderness.

## URODYNAMICS IN PRACTICE: THE CONTRACTED BLADDER

- The most striking urodynamic feature is the reduction in first sensation volume and bladder capacity
- Infiltration of the detrusor muscle by fibrosis or carcinoma reduces the compliance of the bladder so that in most cases there is an inappropriate and linear pressure rise during filling
- In some cases fibrosis around the bladder neck prevents closure and so leads to incontinence during filling associated with a hypocompliant pressure rise as well as stress incontinence
- In a similar way fibrosis around the ureteric orifices may cause vesicoureteral reflux
- In cases of severe bladder contracture the upper tracts act as a reservoir for urine, holding far more than the bladder (Figure 3.10C(ii))
- In addition to causing hypocompliance during filling, fibrosis of the detrusor muscle layer will also reduce the efficiency of the detrusor during voiding, so resulting in detrusor underactivity with reduction of the voiding pressure and sometimes compensatory voiding straining
- Best assessed by videocystometrography (Figure 7.1)
- On fluoroscopy the bladder is commonly noted to be unusually spherical. Incontinence and vesicoureteral reflux may be noted during filling
- Because the contracted bladder is thick-walled and the efficiency of the detrusor may be impaired emptying may be incomplete

## Management

Bladder contracture is the end-stage of treatment for carcinoma by radiotherapy and chronic inflammatory disorders of the bladder. In most cases treatment will have already failed to halt disease progression and therefore operative treatment is indicated. Most cases of contracture due to bladder carcinoma are best treated by cystectomy and urinary diversion or bladder reconstruction.

Dimethyl sulphoxide softens collagen, but intravesical instillation of this agent in cases of bladder contracture due to chronic interstitial cystitis has not been shown to have a lasting beneficial effect.

Cystodistension under general anaesthetic does not produce long-term symptomatic relief.

Most severe cases of fibrotic bladder contracture ultimately require substitution cystoplasty. The details of this is beyond the scope of this book. However, subtotal cystectomy and bladder replacement with ileum are the most widely used operations.

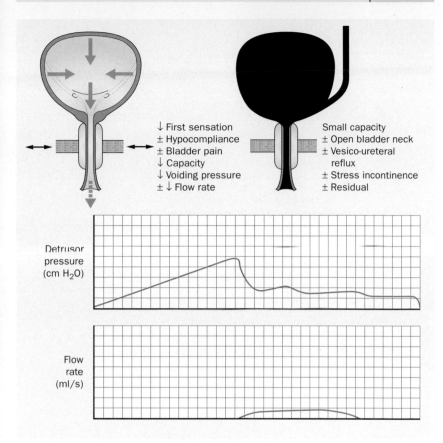

↓ First sensation
± Hypocompliance
± Bladder pain
↓ Capacity
↓ Voiding pressure
± ↓ Flow rate

Small capacity
± Open bladder neck
± Vesico-ureteral
  reflux
± Stress incontinence
± Residual

Detrusor
pressure
(cm H₂O)

Flow
rate
(ml/s)

**Figure 7.1   Typical cystometrogram and videocystometrogram appearances for a contracted bladder.**

# Chapter 8 | Neuropathic Bladder

## INTRODUCTION

Neuropathic bladder dysfunction describes abnormal function of the bladder and urethra due to lesions affecting their innervation, either within the central nervous system or in the peripheral nerves of the lower urinary tract. Vesiocourethral dysfunction is a common feature of many systemic and local neurological conditions.

Urodynamic investigations characterize the nature of the detrusor and sphincteric abnormality to:

- identify those patients who are at risk of deteriorating renal function as a result of the abnormally high bladder pressures; and
- formulate the best treatment strategies to achieve efficient bladder emptying and continence and reduce the incidence of urinary tract infections and autonomic dysreflexia.

The interpretation of urodynamics in such complex cases is often difficult and is best performed in specialist centres using videocystometography (VCMG).

Neurological conditions can alter vesicourethral function by impairing:

- detrusor activity;
- striated sphincter activity;
- bladder and urethral sensation; and
- urethral smooth muscle activity.

These alterations may occur in isolation or in combination. Identical abnormalities may also occur without clinical evidence of a neurological deficit.

### Types of altered vesicourethral function
#### Absent or diminished detrusor activity
Detrusor activity may be absent or diminished if there are lesions of the cell bodies or parasympathetic efferents to the bladder from the sacral roots (S2–S4). This may be due to:

- trauma to the spinal cord or pelvic nerves; or
- destruction of the cord segment by lesions such as a plaque of multiple sclerosis.

### Detrusor overactivity (hyperreflexia)

This may result if there is damage above the level of the sacral cord leading to loss of voluntary control of the detrusor. This may be due to:

- myelomeningocoele;
- cerebrovascular haemorrhage or thrombosis;
- trauma;
- multiple sclerosis;
- tumour; or
- other neurological diseases.

Detrusor contractions may be spontaneous or provoked by bladder filling (as in the 'automatic bladder').

### Detrusor–sphincter dyssynergia

The striated muscle element of the distal urethral sphincter mechanism may fail to relax during voiding. This is detrusor–sphincter dyssynergia and results from suprasacral lesions (see p. 136).

Weakness of the striated sphincter muscle may occur with lesions distal to or including its sacral nerve supply.

The smooth muscle element of the urethral sphincter mechanism may also be disturbed with neurological lesions.

### Loss of sensation within the bladder or urethra

This may occur after local damage to pelvic nerves or the spinal cord.

## Interpretation of vesicourethral dysfunction

Because so many different aspects of vesicourethral function can be impaired in neurological conditions interpretation may be difficult. The most important points to clarify in clinical practice are:

- the presence or absence of detrusor hyperreflexia; and
- the behaviour of the distal urethral sphincter mechanism during voiding.

High-pressure bladders with detrusor–sphincter dyssynergia are prone to develop vesicoureteral reflux, which may ultimately lead to renal impairment. This can be clearly demonstrated by VCMG. Preservation of renal function is of utmost importance in the management of patients who have chronic neurological conditions. As a rule of thumb those patients with a competent bladder outflow and an end filling pressure of 40 cm $H_2O$ or higher are at particular risk of developing upper urinary tract problems due to backpressure.

## Management

Detrusor hyperreflexia in isolation can be treated in the same way as detrusor instability (see Chapter 4).

Detrusor–sphincter dyssynergia may require operative treatment to the sphincter in the form of sphincterotomy or permanently implanted stent insertion and the incontinence that should result from these procedures can be controlled by implanting an artificial urinary sphincter (e.g. the Brantley Scott prosthesis).

## Classification of neuropathic bladder dysfunction

Neuropathic bladder dysfunction may be classified into supraspinal, suprasacral, and infrasacral, according to the level of the lesion in relation to the pontine and sacral micturition centres:

- supraspinal lesions include all cerebral diseases such as cerebral haemorrhage and thrombosis, dementia, tumours, arteriosclerosis, and Parkinson's disease;
- suprasacral lesions are all spinal cord lesions above the conus; and
- infrasacral lesions involve the conus or sacral roots and may be further subdivided into cauda equina lesions (within the spinal canal) and peripheral lesions (outside the spinal canal).

Neurological lesions generally affect bladder and urethral function in a relatively consistent fashion, depending upon the area affected and the completeness of the lesion. A basic understanding of the bladder dysfunction associated with each level of injury is necessary to interpret the results of urodynamics properly.

### Supraspinal lesions

Supraspinal neuropathic bladder dysfunction is characterized by detrusor hyperreflexia associated with coordinated detrusor–sphincter function. The Standardisation Committee of the International Continence Society defines detrusor hyperreflexia as uninhibited detrusor contractions occurring in association with an underlying neurological cause (Figure 8.1).

With supraspinal lesions the bladder hyperactivity is due to absence of cerebral inhibition of the micturition reflex, which is governed by the pontine micturition centre. Similarly, an intact pons ensures coordination of external sphincter activity with detrusor contractions.

The most common symptoms are:

- urinary frequency;
- nocturia; and
- urgency (and even urge incontinence).

Unconscious incontinence occurs when the ascending sensory pathways are disrupted, usually because the resultant sensory damage leads to retention with overflow.

Patients who have supraspinal lesions generally empty their bladders efficiently unless they have associated bladder outlet obstruction. Pre-existing bladder dysfunction is not uncommon and urodynamics plays a major role in defining the abnormality and formulating treatment strategies.

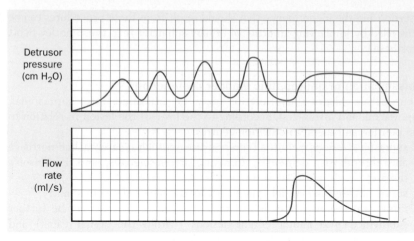

**Figure 8.1  Cystometrogram of detrusor hyperreflexia.** Note the relatively low voiding pressure and 'normal' flow rate.

Supraspinal lesions are often associated with a period of spinal shock and urinary retention, but the bladder generally recovers much more rapidly than with spinal cord lesions.

### Suprasacral lesions

Patients who have cord lesions above the sacral micturition centre initially go through a period of spinal shock in which there is loss of neurological activity below the level of the injury. Detrusor areflexia (the inability to generate a detrusor contraction due to neurological causes) and maintenance of some residual sphincteric competence usually results in urinary retention requiring either indwelling or intermittent catheterization.

Recovery is characterized by the gradual return of reflex bladder activity or detrusor hyperreflexia mediated through the sacral micturition centre, which is intact but separated from higher centres. It usually occurs within 2–3 months, but in a small number of patients it may take up to 2 years for reflex activity to return.

As reflex bladder activity increases during the recovery phase, the bladder may empty well at the expense of incontinence or high detrusor voiding pressures may develop resulting in hydronephrosis.

Inefficient bladder emptying may result from poorly sustained detrusor contractions or detrusor–sphincter dyssynergia (DSD, see Figure 4.5, p. 88), which is involuntary contraction of the external sphincter during a voiding contraction and is highly suggestive of a neurological disorder.

In most cases of DSD, electromyographic (EMG) activity increases during detrusor contraction. DSD occurs in approximately 70–100% of patients who have suprasacral cord lesions following spinal cord injury.

*Infrasacral lesions*

Injury to the conus or sacral roots results in:

- detrusor areflexia;
- a denervated open bladder neck;
- a paralysed closed external sphincter; and
- in most patients, urinary retention.

The weakened urethral sphincter mechanism and paralysed pelvic floor make patients prone to stress incontinence, especially women.

Some patients empty their bladders by abdominal straining or suprapubic compression (Credé's manoeuvre), but the majority need clean intermittent self-catheterization to empty efficiently. For poorly understood reasons, a minority of patients are at risk of developing poorly compliant high-pressure bladders that can lead to renal damage.

Partial infrasacral lesions may result in a mixed pattern of weak or absent detrusor activity, poor compliance, and considerable reflex activity in the pelvic floor muscles.

## URODYNAMICS IN PRACTICE: NEUROPATHIC BLADDER DYSFUNCTION

- Initial urodynamic study is most commonly performed 3–4 months after spinal cord injury when reflex detrusor activity is re-established, along with a baseline renal ultrasound or intravenous urography
- Routine urodynamics and renal radiography are usually performed annually or every alternate year depending upon the nature of the vesicourethral dysfunction and the practice of the treating urologist
- Indications for subsequent urodynamic investigation in spinal cord patients and patients who have other underlying neurological disorders include symptomatic voiding dysfunction, urinary incontinence, renal deterioration (renal scarring, hydronephrosis, elevated serum creatinine), recurrent urinary tract infections, a change in voiding pattern, and the onset of autonomic dysreflexia

**Technique**
- Paralysed patients unable to stand are studied in the supine oblique position to obtain maximal visualization of the bladder neck and urethra
- Voided urine can be transferred from the patient to the flowmeter using a length of polythene drainpipe, which is fixed to the penis and thigh with tape
- Many authorities recommend not emptying the bladder before starting the cystometrogram (CMG) in patients who have detrusor hyperreflexia because these people have persistently high residual urine and rapid bladder evacuation may alter the incidence and characteristics of

detrusor hyperreflexia and result in an overdiagnosis of poor bladder compliance

- Residual urine estimation by catheter or ultrasound should be obtained at another time when emptying is more physiological
- Some patients can improve emptying during urodynamics by abdominal straining, Credé's manoeuvre, or triggering reflex detrusor contractions by perineal or abdominal tapping.
- Although filling rates have been standardized as slow, medium, and fast fill by the International Continence Society Committee, recommendations for filling rates for neuropathic bladder patients vary – for patients who have hyperactive detrusors a fill rate that is too fast may cause early detrusor hyperreflexia, potentially masking information regarding sensation, capacity, and compliance; unphysiological rapid filling rates may also trigger detrusor–sphincter dyssynergia as well as overdiagnose poor bladder compliance; most authors recommend a filling rate of 20–30 ml/min and to allow 30 s at the end of filling for bladder accommodation before interpreting end filling pressure
- Observation of several voiding sequences is recommended to accurately define bladder and urethral abnormalities – the first voiding sequence may be altered by passing the catheter, which may precipitate or inhibit detrusor hyperreflexia and be unrepresentative of the established pattern; suprapubic catheterization may eliminate this problem and is routinely used by some spinal cord centres
- Symptomatic urinary tract infections alter urodynamic results and should be treated before urodynamic evaluation – asymptomatic bacteriuria is common and predisposes patients to bacteraemia; it is recommended to use parenteral antibiotics 1 hour before study
- Videourodynamics provides state-of-the-art evaluation of patients who have neuropathic bladder dysfunction. Radiographic contrast medium used during videourodynamics has the advantages of fluid cystometry while allowing simultaneous anatomical characterization of the bladder and urethra. Providing information about bladder size and shape, the presence of vesicoureteral reflux, the competency of the bladder neck, and the site of bladder outflow obstruction; it diminishes the importance of simultaneous electromyography for diagnosing detrusor–sphincter dyssynergia; poor fluoroscopic visualization of the bladder secondary to a high initial residual urine volume, obesity, or constipation is not uncommon and to provide adequate visualization, a small volume of 50% contrast medium should be added to the filling medium.

## Practical points

Performing urodynamics in patients who have neuropathic bladder dysfunction can be challenging, and technique modifications may be necessary to obtain the maximum amount of information. Sudden bursts of leg or abdominal spasms are not uncommon and may precede detrusor reflex contractions or result in loss of the recording catheters.

Rectal impaction can theorectically alter vesicourethral function during urodynamic evaluation and rectal evacuation before study is advised. If suppositories or rectal solutions are used, urodynamics should be delayed until there is a bowel action. Rectal catheterization commonly stimulates bowel evacuation in patients who have a spinal cord injury.

The type of catheter used is the same as for non-neurological cases, but transurethral catheterization may be difficult in patients who have suprasacral cord lesions because of external sphincter muscle spasm.

### Autonomic dysreflexia

Autonomic dysreflexia is the exaggerated sympathetic output that occurs in response to a noxious stimulus below the level of injury in patients who have spinal cord injuries above T6. Bladder overdistension or high detrusor pressures may precipitate episodes of hypertension associated with bradycardia, headache, and profuse sweating and flushing above the level of the injury. Similarly, urodynamics can precipitate autonomic dysreflexia during filling or in relation to detrusor–sphincter dyssynergia and can be instrumental in helping with the diagnosis.

If autonomic dysreflexia occurs during urodynamic studies bladder filling should be stopped and the bladder emptied and sublingual nifedipine 10 mg may be needed to treat the hypertension. Provocation of dysreflexia during urodynamic evaluation may be prevented by slow filling rates, maintenance of low volumes and detrusor pressures, and oral chlorpromazine before study.

# ELECTROMYOGRAPHY

Electromyography (see pp. 67–69) is the study of the bioelectric potentials generated by depolarization of skeletal muscle and here this refers to the distal striated urethral sphincter mechanism. The primary value of EMG is for identifying neuropathy. The functional unit in EMG is the motor unit, which is comprised of:
- a varying number of muscle fibres supplied by the same motor neurone originating as an anterior horn cell; and
- the axon of the motor neurone.

An excitory impulse in the motor neurone causes each of its muscle fibres to contract and the summated activity from the synchronously activated muscle fibres in the motor unit is called the motor unit action potential (MUAP). The waveform of the MUAP is generally biphasic or triphasic and may be detected by electrodes and displayed on an oscilloscope screen or strip chart. Individually recorded on an oscilloscope, the MUAP has its own amplitude, duration, and firing frequency.

When a motor neurone is damaged the muscle fibres that have lost their nerve supply become reinnervated by adjacent healthy nerve fibres by a process called collateral sprouting, resulting in fewer but larger motor units. This results in MUAPs of larger amplitude and increased complexity (polyphasic) and duration. These changes in EMG may be used to infer the presence of neurological disease.

## Types of electrodes
### Surface electrodes
Surface electrodes (skin, anal plug, catheter) record total electrical output from the neighbouring muscles of the pelvic floor and are the standard electrodes used in clinical practice. They cannot record individual MUAPs, but allow assessment of overall muscle behaviour, which is recorded directly onto a paper chart strip recorder or recorded as sound through an audio monitor.

Surface electrodes should be applied to the epithelium as close to the muscle under study as possible. They can be difficult to secure and provide less reproducible results than needle electrodes.

### Needle electrodes
Individual MUAPs may be detected by needle electrodes placed directly into or near the muscle to be studied and displayed on an oscilloscope screen. Most commonly the needle is placed directly into the periurethral sphincter. A variety of different types of needle electrodes exist including concentric, bipolar, monopolar, and single fibre.

Needle electrodes permit a more precise recording of EMG activity and analysis of individual MUAPs than surface electrodes. The technique is, however, user-dependent and requires considerable expertise. Its use is therefore generally limited to research and highly specialized centres.

## Recording site
An EMG can be recorded from three muscles:
- external anal sphincter;
- levator ani; and
- intrinsic striated urethral sphincter.

The easiest muscle to use is the external anal sphincter because placement is simple and dislodgement is less common.

In most patients the EMG recorded from the three sites is similar, but in some neurological disorders, particularly demyelinating disease and partial cauda equina lesions, there may be significant differences between the recordings. It is therefore recommended by many to always record from the periurethral musculature.

### Interpretation

Volitional control of the urinary sphincter is demonstrated by an increase and decrease in EMG activity associated with active contraction and relaxation of the pelvic floor musculature respectively. During filling there is a normal progressive increase in EMG activity referred to as recruitment. Electrical silence during EMG measurement should precede the onset of voiding and persist throughout the detrusor contraction. Persistent EMG activity during voiding can be due to:

- the fact that complete electrical silence does not always occur;
- straining artefact;
- detrusor–sphincter dyssynergia; and
- pseudodyssynergia.

Pseudodyssynergia is the normal voluntary contraction of the external sphincter and pelvic floor muscles in response to an uninhibited detrusor contraction in an attempt to prevent urge incontinence.

True detrusor–sphincter dyssynergia occurs only in patients who have neurological disorders and ranges in severity from active contraction to failure of relaxation of the external sphincter during voiding contractions.

## SPECIALIZED NEUROPHYSIOLOGICAL STUDIES

### Nerve conduction studies

These are performed by stimulating a peripheral nerve and monitoring the time for a response to occur in its innervated muscle. The time from stimulation of a motor nerve to the first measurable muscle response is termed the motor latency.

Latency studies test the integrity of nerve pathways, demonstrating prolonged latencies when there is injury to the nerve with associated demyelination. The most commonly tested latency used to assess neuropathic bladder dysfunction is the bulbocavernosus reflex.

Nerve conduction studies are a beneficial tool in diagnosing neurological disease, but require elaborate instrumentation and expert interpretation.

### Evoked responses

Evoked responses are potential changes in neural tissue resulting from distant stimulation, usually electrical. They are used to test the integrity of peripheral, spinal, and central nervous pathways. As with nerve conduction studies, their usage is confined to specialized neurophysiology centres.

## SPECIALIZED TESTING

### Bethanechol supersensitivity test

The bethanechol supersensitivity test is based on Cannon's law of denervation, which states that when an organ is deprived of its nerve supply it will develop hypersensitivity to its own neurotransmitter.

A 2.5 mg dose of bethanechol chloride, an acetylcholine-like parasympathomimetic agent, is administered subcutaneously following an initial CMG. During repeat CMG, a rise in pressure of more than 15 cm $H_2O$ difference at 100 ml filling is a positive result and implies detrusor denervation.

False negative and false postive results are common and bethanechol is contraindicated for patients who have cardiac disease, hypertension, asthma, peptic ulcer, or bladder outlet obstruction.

Although of limited use, the bethanechol supersensitvity test may prove beneficial in differentiating myogenic from neuropathic detrusor acontractility.

### Ice water test

The ice water test helps differentiate between detrusor hyperreflexia and areflexia following spinal cord injury.

The test is performed by instilling 90 ml of sterile ice-cold water (4°C) into an empty bladder through a 16 F catheter without filling the balloon.

The test is positive for detrusor hyperreflexia if the catheter is ejected together with a significant amount of water within 1 min in the absence of straining.

The technique can be modified by using ice water provocation during cystometry to stimulate reflex detrusor activity.

## AMBULATORY URODYNAMICS

Conventional pressure–flow urodynamics form the cornerstone of an understanding of neuropathic bladder dysfunction. Disadvantages of conventional studies include:

- nonphysiological filling rates; and
- relatively short testing periods.

Ambulatory urodynamics allows long-term bladder monitoring under more normal circumstances while the bladder is filled at a physiological rate and may have an application for patients who have neurological disease. It has been shown that elevated bladder pressure demonstrated by conventional filling cystometry may significantly lessen during ambulatory studies. Ambulatory urodynamics at present is considered to be a research tool.

# Chapter 9 | Paediatric urodynamics

Paediatric urodynamics has become a specialized field with the development of child-oriented techniques and better understanding of both non-neuropathic and neuropathic bladder dysfunction in children.

As a general rule, urodynamics is not routinely required in the evaluation of non-neuropathic paediatric voiding dysfunction because in most cases adequate diagnosis and treatment can be based upon a thorough history and physical examination, and appropriate use of endoscopy and radiography.

Most paediatric urological cases are well-recognised functional voiding disorders or have an underlying abnormality such as bladder outlet obstruction and diagnosis does not depend upon the use of urodynamics. However, urodynamic studies are the mainstay investigations in the evaluation and treatment of children with neuropathic bladder dysfunction, which is most commonly due to spinal abnormalities.

## INDICATIONS FOR URODYNAMICS

In the absence of neurological disease, indications for urodynamic investigations in children include:
- voiding dysfunction associated with significant bladder hypertrophy, vesicoureteral reflux, or upper urinary tract damage;
- diurnal incontinence that is troublesome for the child, refractory to conservative therapy, and is not typical of common functional voiding disorders;
- symptomatic patients suspected of having occult neuropathy; and
- rarely, some children who have persistent nocturnal enuresis and recurrent urinary tract infections.

## HISTORY AND EXAMINATION

Before proceeding with urodynamics a detailed history and physical examination are required to:
- characterize the bladder dysfunction;
- look for underlying organic disease; and
- identify common functional voiding syndromes.

A detailed voiding history is essential and should include:
- age and results of toilet training;

- occurrence of primary or secondary enuresis;
- specific pattern of wetting, such as stress incontinence, continual dripping, or urge incontinence;
- manoeuvres used to prevent wetting such as squatting; and
- frequency of daytime and night-time micturition.

Physical examination should include:
- inspection of the genitalia;
- palpation of the lumbosacral spine to detect vertebral defects or sacral agenesis;
- examination of the skin overlying the spine for hairy patches, dimples, or bumps that might indicate occult spinal abnormalities;
- inspection of the lower extremities for subtle neuropathy-related bony abnormalities; and
- a careful sensorimotor neurological examination.

The most common functional voiding disorder in children is idiopathic primary bladder instability or immature bladder syndrome, which is common in 4- to 7-year-olds. Symptoms commonly include frequency and urge incontinence, and bladder signals appear to be ignored during play activities. Girls may display the Vincent's curtsey sign where the heel is pressed into the perineum to prevent incontinence secondary to unstable bladder contractions.

Most cases resolve spontaneously, but a number may require a period of anticholinergic medication to alleviate the symptoms. Urodynamic studies add little to the diagnosis and treatment of these children and should be reserved for selected cases.

## URODYNAMICS IN PRACTICE: PAEDIATRIC PATIENTS

- Urodynamics in children requires time, patience, and above all, experienced interpretation

### Uroflowmetry
- In general the usefulness of uroflowmetry in the evaluation of paediatric voiding dysfunction is limited – flow rates vary with age, sex, and volume voided, preventing the establishment of standard values
- Uroflowmetry requires that the child is old enough to follow instructions and void in his or her usual fashion – a normal pattern associated with efficient bladder emptying may be sufficient, making further urodynamic testing unnecessary
- A straining pattern may be identified during uroflowmetry or diagnosed by the simultaneous recording of pelvic floor or abdominal skeletal muscle electromyography (EMG)

## Cystometry
- Water cystometry is recommended using 5–8 F urethral catheters or feeding tubes
- There may be a role for suprapubic catheterization in selected patients
- Infusion rates depend upon the age of the child and therefore bladder capacity – it is normal to fill adults at the rate of 10–20% of expected bladder capacity/min (i.e. 50–100 ml/min) and we use the same ratio principle for children; markedly lower rates should be used for cases of neuropathic bladder
- Simultaneous measurement of intra-abdominal pressure should be recorded by rectal catheterization – if the rectal catheter is not well tolerated, abdominal wall EMG may be used to detect abdominal wall muscle activity, giving an indirect measure of abdominal pressure; in many cases the pressure/filling catheter is inserted suprapubically preoperatively under anaesthetic
- The bladder is filled with the patient supine using standard provocative manoeuvres and the child is encouraged to void in a position and fashion that are as normal as possible
- Children should be fully awake during cystometry, but in some cases mild sedation is required to obtain useful information

## Electromyography
- Electromyography of the striated muscles of the pelvic floor is necessary to assess synergy between the bladder and urethral sphincter mechanisms during voiding
- Surface patch electrodes are used in most cases, but fine needle electrodes placed directly into the periurethral striated sphincter are recommended to diagnose neuropathy, but this is not normally feasible in children
- Increased EMG activity secondary to straining is common in children and must be differentiated from true detrusor–sphincter dyssynergia, which is diagnostic of neuropathic bladder dysfunction

## Urethral pressure profile
- Urethral pressure profile studies are of limited value in paediatric urodynamics as children will not tolerate the urethral discomfort sometimes associated with the study

## Videourodynamics
- Videourodynamics provides a more comprehensive evaluation, especially in patients who have neuropathic bladder dysfunction, bladder outlet obstruction, and incontinence
- Detrusor–sphincter dyssynergia can be diagnosed during fluoroscopy without direct measurement of EMG activity, eliminating the need for potentially bothersome electrodes

## Practical points

Patient cooperation, as well as reproduction of the child's normal voiding pattern, is of utmost importance to obtain useful clinical information. A pleasant cheerful testing environment and staff, and the presence of a family member, help reduce patient fear and anxiety. Common helpful distractors include video, television, games, toys, and favourite treats.

## Interpretation

It is likely that all children transiently display abnormalities in bladder and sphincter function when making the transition from infantile to adult patterns of urinary control. Provided that these are neither sustained nor repetitive, they do not appear to be pathological or to carry any long-term consequences. Because of the great variability in the way that young children develop urinary control, extreme caution is needed in interpreting their urodynamics and in diagnosing disorders of vesicourethral function. Urodynamics must therefore not be undertaken lightly in this age group.

Cystometry provides useful information about bladder capacity, sensation, compliance, and stability. The maximum cystometric capacity is often lower than the calculated anatomical capacity and depends upon the child's ability to suppress voiding. Filling is usually limited by:

- a sensation of bladder fullness or even pain;
- urinary incontinence secondary to bladder instability or poor detrusor compliance; or
- uncontrollable spontaneous voiding.

An estimation of bladder sensitivity (hypersensitive, hyposensitive, or normal) can be made during filling.

Bladder instability may or may not represent a clinically significant abnormality, depending upon the patient's age and voluntary response to it. Unstable contractions are considered to be normal in young immature bladders until central inhibitory pathways develop to produce detrusor stability, even in the face of a strong desire to void. This usually occurs by 4 years of age, and often much sooner. Voiding is involuntary and usually to completion as a result of a well-sustained detrusor contraction accompanied by synergic relaxation of the urethral sphincter mechanism.

Voluntary contraction of the external sphincter in an attempt to prevent incontinence is common in the early development of normal urinary control. This results in an obstruction to flow with high intravesical pressure. In some children, this voluntary dyssynergia can remain, resulting in long-term voiding dysfunction. Renal damage can result in the most severe cases and this group can be labelled as non-neuropathic neuropathic bladder or Hinman's syndrome.

Voluntary contraction of the external sphincter to prevent leakage during unstable bladder contractions is commonly misinterpreted as detrusor–sphincter dyssynergia in patients who do not have neuropathy. This is an appropriate patient response in an attempt to maintain continence and is properly referred to as pseudodyssynergia. To make this important distinction, the external sphincter relaxes and EMG activity becomes silent in normal asymptomatic controls when the patient is asked to void voluntarily.

Reduced bladder compliance is commonly found in patients who have neuropathic bladder dysfunction. End filling pressure is normally below 10 cm $H_2O$. Children who have myelomeningocoele and reduced bladder compliance with a detrusor leak point pressure over 40 cm $H_2O$ are at risk of renal damage as a result of the high detrusor pressure.

Urodynamics plays an important role in the identification of patients at risk of renal damage and provides the physician with an objective measure for assessing treatment efficacy.

To date, there are limited ambulatory urodynamic data for patients who have neuropathic bladder and although early results have yielded interesting findings its clinical role has not yet been established.

# Chapter 10 | Lower urinary tract symptoms in pregnancy

## INTRODUCTION

Lower urinary tract symptoms (LUTS) are common in pregnancy. Most studies of the lower urinary tract in pregnancy have in the past concentrated on the prevalence of abnormal voiding patterns and incontinence in very general terms. Only recently have more specific reports reviewed individual symptoms including urgency, urge incontinence, and voiding difficulties.

## VOIDING PATTERNS

There are no standardized definitions of voiding patterns in pregnancy, which makes studies difficult to compare.

Increased frequency of micturition and nocturia are very common in pregnancy (80% of pregnant women) and tend to worsen as the pregnancy progresses. These are multifactorial in origin and causes include:

- pressure of the gravid uterus on the bladder producing a change in bladder capacity;
- altered urine production and biochemistry; and
- an increased number of hours spent resting.

It is also likely that there are as yet unidentified other aspects including systemic hormonal influences and local tissue effects. Those women who experience the greatest increase in frequency both during the day and at night are less likely to return to their pre-pregnancy state. This suggests that the changes seen may be structural, but it is likely that there is also a marked contributory behavioural component.

## INCONTINENCE

Women who have severe stress or urge incontinence during pregnancy are more likely to continue to experience this postnatally than women who have less severe stress or urge incontinence during pregnancy.

### Stress incontinence
Stress incontinence is a symptom, a sign, and a condition, but not a specific diagnosis – the qualification of 'genuine' stress incontinence represents a diagnosis based on urodynamic assessment.

Stress incontinence is common in pregnancy, but is generally a transient symptom with only a small proportion of women remaining incontinent long term. There is still considerable debate about which component of pregnancy – labour or delivery – causes it (Figure 10.1).

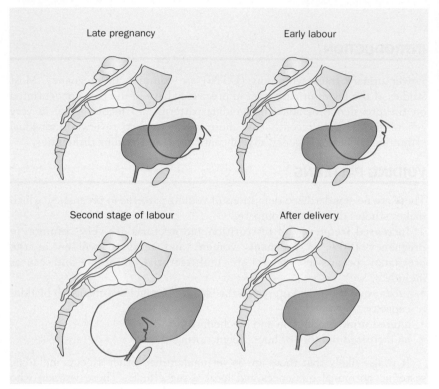

**Figure 10.1 Movement of the bladder in late pregnancy and during and after delivery.**

### Urge incontinence

Urgency and urge incontinence commonly occur *de novo* during pregnancy and usually resolve postpartum. Conversely the symptoms of some women who have sensory disorders of the urinary tract resolve during pregnancy; LUTS occurring as a consequence of endometriosis usually improve.

### Causes

Lower urinary tract symptoms and function correlate poorly with urodynamic diagnoses in nonpregnant woman, and this lack of agreement has also been shown in pregnancy. It is unclear what the precise contribution of the individual components of pregnancy, labour, and delivery is in the genesis of lower urinary tract dysfunction in any individual, particularly as it is usually a retrospective diagnosis.

Changes in the position of the bladder neck shown radiologically during labour result in stretching of supporting structures, leading to damage and weakening of urethral sphincter mechanisms.

Soft tissues in pregnancy have a reduced tensile strength (due to hormonal influences), which may account for the development of stress incontinence in pregnancy. Although postpartum the fascia will regain its previous strength, it may be that it has already undergone irreversible damage by overstretching in cases with established stress incontinence.

Electromyography has been used to examine the effects of vaginal delivery on denervation of the sphincter mechanism. It appears that pelvic floor denervation occurs more commonly in women who undergo a vaginal delivery than in those undergoing a caesarean section.

The major factor in labour associated with sphincter damage is thought to be a prolonged first stage and a long-duration active (pushing) second stage. It can therefore be argued that a trial of 'normal' labour should be time-limited, particularly in primiparous women. There is a lower prevalence of stress incontinence in women who have a forceps delivery under epidural analgesia than among those who have a pudendal block. It has been suggested that an epidural may protect the pelvic floor during delivery by enabling it to relax during delivery. Furthermore, cystometry studies have confirmed that the prevalence of detrusor instability is significantly greater antenatally than postpartum.

Urinary incontinence in pregnancy and the postpartum period may be due to different pathological processes, with detrusor instability predominating as an aetiological factor during pregnancy, and sphincteric weakness becoming more important in the postpuerperal urinary tract.

### Prevention and management

If antenatal LUTS are physiological and have no long-term sequelae, then reassurance is all that is required. However, these transient symptoms could be a marker for long-term sequelae and it is difficult to forecast their true significance in an individual case.

An elective caesarean section should be advised for 'at risk' women (i.e. women who have undergone an effective incontinence procedure before pregnancy).

A simple noninvasive preventive measure may be formal teaching of pelvic floor exercises, before the pelvic floor has been damaged. This can be coordinated through family planning clinics, sex education lessons, and pre-pregnancy counselling clinics. If the muscle is already damaged, pelvic floor training is unlikely to be effective.

Anticholinergic therapy for detrusor instability in pregnancy cannot be justified because of potential toxicity to the fetus and associated side effects to the patient. Incontinence persisting postnatally should be investigated.

## STORAGE DISORDERS

Most cases of incontinence are transient and investigation can be delayed until at least 6 weeks postpartum. However, if the patient complains of the continuous leakage of urine, investigation is mandatory to exclude retention with overflow or a urinary fistula.

Symptoms of apparent storage difficulty appear to be fairly common in pregnancy. These usually result in small volumes of urine being passed at frequent intervals as a result of the:

- reduced capacity of the bladder (extravesical compression); and
- increased pressure on the urethral sphincter mechanism.

Not surprisingly, the impact of preexisting disorders of detrusor function such as detrusor instability may become more pronounced.

## VOIDING DISORDERS

Urinary retention in pregnancy is uncommon and usually results from an impacted retroverted uterus at about 16 weeks of gestation. It probably results from interference with the normal opening of the bladder outlet due to the enlarged uterus.

Treatment is bladder drainage (intermittent self-catheterization) and manual correction of the uterus into a more anteverted position using a ring pessary.

Investigation of any associated detrusor malfunction is delayed to postpartum and is usually reserved for those patients who have either large postvoiding residual urine volumes or continuing symptoms.

It is now well established that after epidural analgesia, the bladder takes up to 8 hours to regain its sensation and within this time period the bladder must be adequately drained. If not, the subsequent overdistension of the bladder may result in detrusor damage and if undetected may result in long-term voiding difficulties. Attention should be paid to those patients at risk of developing retention, in particular those who have had:

- traumatic delivery;
- prolonged labour;
- epidural analgesia;
- caesarean section; or
- previous voiding problems at any time especially after previous deliveries.

Voiding alone should not be accepted at face value and even input–output charts can be misleading. It is therefore important to check postvoiding residual volume. Ideally an indwelling urethral catheter should be inserted and left for up to 12 hours following an epidural or caesarean section and after other 'high risk' deliveries.

It is clear that there are a number of areas where present knowledge is extremely rudimentary and where urodynamic investigation will help us understand more about normal function and the pathophysiology of the lower urinary tract both during pregnancy and postpartum.

## FURTHER READING

Abrams P. Urodynamics, 2nd ed. London: Springer-Verlag; 1997.

Abrams P, Griffiths D, Buzelin JM, *et al*. The urodynamic assessment of lower urinary tract symptoms. In: Denis L, Griffiths K, Khoury S, *et al.*, eds. 4th International Consultation on BPH, Proceedings. Plymouth: Health Publication; 1998:325.

Andersson K-E, Appell R, Cardozo L, *et al*. Pharmacological treatment of urinary incontinence. In: Abrams P, Khoury S, Wein A, eds. 1st International Consultation on Incontinence, Proceedings. Co-sponsored by WHO and International Union Against Cancer. Plymouth: Health Publication; 1999.

Mundy AR, Stephenson TP, Wein AJ, eds. Urodynamics – principles, practice and application, 2nd ed. Edinburgh: Churchill Livingstone; 1994.

# Index